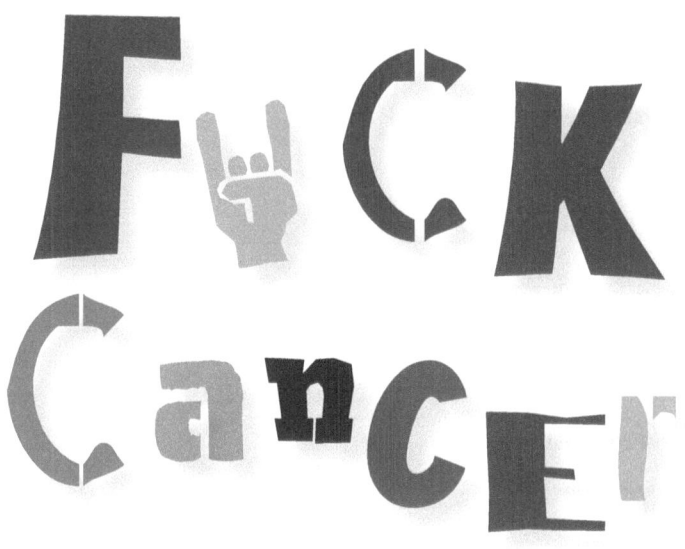

My Story—Blowups with Bryan Adams, Breakouts in Production, and Battles with Cancer

Jonathan Schwartz

Grumpy Press

Copyright © 2025 by Jonathan Schwartz
All rights reserved. No part of this book may be used or reproduced in any manner whatsoever without written permission except in the case of brief quotations embodied in critical articles or reviews.

Published by Grumpy Press

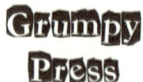

Produced by GMK Writing and Editing, Inc.
Managing Editor: Katie Benoit
Copyedited by Amy Paradysz
Proofread by Elaini Caruso
Text design by Elizabeth Kingsbury
Composition by Joanna Beyer
Cover design by Vicky Vaughn Shea
Printed by IngramSpark

Print ISBN: 978-1-966981-00-8
Ebook EISN: 978-1-966981-01-5

Visit the author at fuckcancerbook.com

Note: This publication is presented solely for informational, educational, and entertainment purposes and is told strictly from the author's point of view and best remembrance of facts. Names of certain individuals have been changed or omitted to protect their right to privacy. To the maximum extent permitted by law, the producer and the author and their affiliated entities and individuals disclaim any and all liability in the event any information contained in this book proves to be inaccurate, incomplete, or unreliable, or results in any harm or loss.

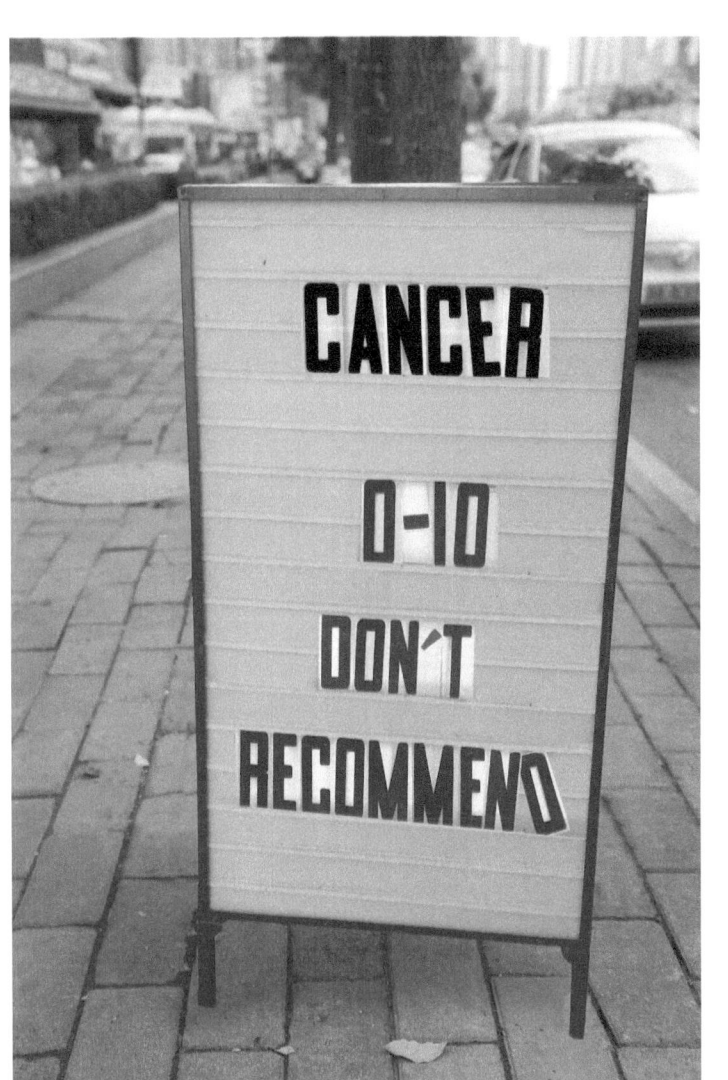

To my rock, Mara.

Acknowledgments

Mara: You are my best friend. My everything. There aren't enough days left to pay you back for all your love and support. I'll forever be grateful.

Alissa and Matt: I think about you all the time. You bring me such happiness. I feel like I won the kid lottery. Love you always.

Smoke and Lacey: You bring me more joy than you will ever know. Dogs are an absolute gift.

Stefanie, my sister: My deepest thanks for not only continuously dispensing nutritional advice but also for being the caring person that you are.

My mother-in-law: Thanks for asking how I'm doing 937 times a day.

Merri: How do I pay you back? When I was stuck in quicksand, you immediately connected me to your friend at Memorial Sloan Kettering Cancer Center and got the ball rolling. Forever thanks.

Bunny and Steve: You've been unbelievably generous with your apartment. When you heard what I was going through, you didn't hesitate to step in and help. I'm so touched.

My work family at Washington Square Films—especially Josh, my partner for over a quarter of a century. I've learned so much from you and am so much of a better person because of you. You are almost always right. The proof is in the countless Academy Award nominations, Sundance films, Cannes awards, Emmy Awards, and other accomplishments. Much respect.

Jeff, Ed, and Keith, my friends since middle school: Nothing replaces best friends. I never thought that when we were stealing Humpty-Dumpty from the eighteenth hole of the mini-golf course in Ocean City that we'd end up here. Your support means everything.

Chris & Jean, Jeff & Lauren, Don & Anne, Ray & Erin, Joel & Erica, and everyone else in the 'hood—my neighbors: When we moved to Stoneleigh Square, I was hoping not to get stuck with the neighbor who lights fireworks off their porch at 4:00 a.m. What we got was literally the greatest neighbors you could ever ask for. Thank you for all the rides, calls, meals, concerts, and everything else. You guys are the best.

Gary & Liz, Scott & Lisa, Eric & Lisa, Mark & Susan, Max, David—my Fairfield friends: Thanks for being such a great support network. The concerts have been memorable. Some people just step it up any time you need it. Grateful.

Debbi, queen of Connect Fairfield: I appreciate your knowing everybody and your willingness to always lend a hand.

Dr. Andrew Zelenetz, Dr. Christian Grommes, Dr. Gunjan Shah, and NP extraordinaire Ashley Ames: You are all the Dream Team.

The countless nurses at MSK: All of you saw me through rough times and we shared many laughs together. I wouldn't have made it through without you.

Team Mara, including friends from IP, Albany, and the K'Tanim family: Thank you for being so kind and supportive to us. It's much appreciated.

My mom, I love you always: You unexpectedly passed away two days after my original diagnosis, which maybe was for the best in terms of timing. I'm so glad you didn't have to see me go through all this.

Contents

Prologue: I WAS A PUNK ROCK KID 1
Introduction: SOMETHING'S UP WITH MY SINUSES 5
Chapter One: I LIVED OFF STOUFFER'S FRENCH BREAD PIZZA 19
Chapter Two: MAY THE SCHWARTZES BE WITH US 28
Chapter Three: MY BEEF WITH BRYAN ADAMS 36
Chapter Four: APPLE SHOOTS DURING THE RECESSION 45
Chapter Five: FIFTY FEET OF CRAP IN THE MONEYBALL ERA 53
Chapter Six: STEPPING OVER BODIES AT THE BOWERY 60
Chapter Seven: THE GIFT OF SCHILLERVISION 67
Chapter Eight: SONIC YOUTH AND THE LAST DAYS OF CBGB 73
Chapter Nine: THE GREEN MONSTER INVADES THIRD AVENUE 78
Chapter Ten: HENRY, BECKHAM, AND A BAG OF LAY'S 84
Chapter Eleven: HEY DOC, I HAVE A BUMP ON MY ASS 88
Chapter Twelve: I THINK I HAVE A HEADACHE 96
Epilogue: LAST—BUT DEFINITELY NOT FINAL—WORDS 106
Photos 111
Sources 120
About the Author: Jonathan Schwartz 125
About Grumpy Press 127

Prologue

I was a Punk Rock Kid

> IF I HAD FIVE MILLION POUNDS, I'D START A RADIO STATION BECAUSE SOMETHING NEEDS TO BE DONE. IT WOULD BE NICE TO TURN ON THE RADIO AND HEAR SOMETHING THAT DIDN'T MAKE YOU FEEL LIKE SMASHING UP THE KITCHEN AND STRANGLING THE CAT.
> —JOE STRUMMER

Who is the worst rock band of all time? I say Led Zeppelin. Did I grab your attention?

Judging by the title of this book alone, I'm sure you've already guessed that I'm going to stir some controversy in this book. I'm a no b.s. guy who has been known to speak his mind, drop more than his share of *f*-bombs, and even shoot down one of the most popular rock groups in history.

Although I'm not a musician or even in the music business, I'm starting off my story by defining myself as a punk rock kid, rather than fully addressing the subject of the book: cancer, my career, or even my family. Why? *It's who I am.* Punk rock was—and *still is*—my world. Music transports me to a different place.

I was raised in Chappaqua, New York, by a divorced mom who was cool and supportive and gave me a long rope. We had the smallest house in an affluent town ruled by preppies. You didn't see a lot of punk rock fans around. As a clueless preteen and teenager in the late 1970s to early 80s wearing way too much denim and my Converse sneakers, I'd often take the Metro-North train into New York City with my friends and live it up at the hottest clubs and theaters. I grew up during a certain historic time and place when punk rock ruled, and these venues were my world, my homes away from home: CBGB, Max's Kansas City, the Ritz, Pier 84, the Bowery Ballroom, and the Beacon Theatre. Afterward, we'd take the last train back to Chappaqua and my mom didn't care, as long as I didn't get in trouble (which only happened once; don't worry, we'll get to that later).

You're probably wondering: Why do I hate Led Zeppelin with such passion when nearly so many people consider them one of the best bands ever? I *loathe* screeching guitars (Jimmy Page), high-pitched howling (Robert Plant), and long, boring solos on any instrument (again Page, plus drummer John Bonham). While we're at it, I despise most classic rock and hard rock, including progressive, psychedelic, heavy metal, and jam. With that in mind, you can toss several others on the dung heap: Van Halen, Kiss, Aerosmith, AC/DC, the Grateful Dead, Deep Purple, the Doors, U2, the Who, Black Sabbath, Yes, Rush, and any lineup that featured Eric Clapton.

Now for the classic rock exceptions. The Beatles were clearly the best band of all time, and I appreciate them, although they were never my main thing. I can see the charismatic, enduring appeal of the Rolling Stones; they've recorded a ton of great songs, and I respect them a lot. I enjoy the Kinks (Ray Davies is such a great songwriter) and the Beach Boys (incredible harmonies); both bands have such deep catalogs of amazing hits.

The common denominator that distinguishes artists and bands such as these and my punk favorites—which we'll cover soon, I promise—from Led Zeppelin and the other shit groups? They were off-the-charts creative, had unbeatable catchy melodies, brilliant musical hooks, solid beats, and exceptional harmonies.

This leads me back to punk rock and the band that I saw more than any other, my sweet spot: the Ramones. I don't know how many times I caught them live back then, but they kicked ass on every occasion. They were unique and mesmerizing with a ton of attitude, although they didn't interact with the audience or say much of anything on stage. Their timeless two- to three-minute songs speak for themselves: "Rockaway Beach," "Beat on the Brat," "I Wanna Be Sedated," "Do You Remember Rock 'n' Roll Radio?" "Pet Sematary," "The KKK Took My Baby Away," and on and on.

My favorite band, though, was the Clash, who had three mind-blowing albums in a row: *London Calling*, *Sandinista!*, and *Combat Rock*. Then there were all the other punk rock greats: the Sex Pistols (obviously a lot more on the dangerous side, which I wasn't), the Pogues, Social Distortion, Hüsker Dü, Pixies, Devo, the Violent Femmes (whose first album was mind-blowing), the B-52s, and the Replacements. I also loved

David Bowie, the Talking Heads, REM, Blondie, Lou Reed, the Police, and Joan Jett, who overlapped with classic rock/new wave/alternative but were innovative, had catchy songs, and didn't do those freaking annoying guitar solos. Neil Young is another exception; the guy is raw and rocks.

It feels so good to have got that out of my system, like all the cancer and the crap that was pumped into my system to destroy it—especially chemo and radiation. It's hard not to get pissed off when you have such a great life and, out of nowhere, you get knocked on your ass with cancer over and over. I would bet everyone who has battled this disease—as well as their family and loved ones—has shouted "Fuck cancer!" aloud or at least thought it at one time or another. Offensive as it might sound to some people, I'm going with *F*ck Cancer* as the title of this book because it fits who I am at heart: a punk rock kid from Chappaqua, New York. If you don't like my honesty—well, you know what you can do with yourself.

One last thing: *fuck Jimi Hendrix*. He's the *second* worst artist ever.

Introduction

Something's Up with My Sinuses

JUNE 2021

I DON'T KNOW WHERE I'M GOING FROM HERE, BUT I PROMISE IT WON'T BE BORING.
—DAVID BOWIE

I've always been a total fucking hypochondriac. Every day, I'd come home from work and say to my wife, "Oh my God, Mara, can you take a look at this mark?" or "I've got this crazy itch here, I should run to the doctor."

Things started to go a bit downhill for me around when I hit fifty. Nothing major, but stuff I had to take care of. My hypochondria worked in my favor, so I was able to notice things right away and nip them in the bud. I had chronic gastrointestinal problems, three hernias, and gallbladder removal surgery. I was on small doses of medication to control my cholesterol and regulate my blood pressure and never had any serious cardiovascular issues, even though I'm not a guy who exercises (big understatement) or eats right (*major* understatement: I'm a meat-and-potatoes kind of guy who *detests* fruits and vegetables).

I became so worried about my health that I invested $2,500 a year in a VIP plan with my doctor. This way, anytime something seemed the least bit off, I could call him and schedule an appointment for the next day.

Before June 2021, I thought I had everything under control in terms of my health. I had strong intuition identifying issues early and a doctor who was at my disposal. In fact, I would go as far as saying that my life was going great. I was happy with my marriage—Mara and I had been together for twenty-seven years—and our twins, Alissa and Matt, were both doing well in college.

My job as managing director at Washington Square Films (WSF) running the commercial production side of the business couldn't have been going better. After a year of the 2020 COVID-19 pandemic shutdown shitstorm and being unable to travel and shoot commercials, things had finally eased up and I was back to commuting to my New York office and gradually resuming work on production sets around the United States and the world. Even though I still had to wear a mask, I loved getting back into my neighborhood in the Bowery—my home away from home—and once again working in my office, sitting at my desk, doing business with my WSF coworkers, and grabbing lunch at my favorite places, like Café Habana on Prince Street.

My old routine had resumed in full force when I noticed that something was up with my sinuses. The right upper cheek around the top of my gums was bothering me. I had a slight cough and thought I might be coming down with a cold or something. Ever the hypochondriac, I made an appointment with an ear, nose, and throat doctor near my house in Fairfield, Connecticut.

The doctor checked out my ears, nose, and throat with an otoscope and then did a deeper dive up my nose with a tube to check out the nasal cavity. It's not pleasant, but at least I would get some peace of mind. He completed the examination and said, "Everything looks perfectly fine, Jon—no worries."

I figured that was satisfactory, although it didn't provide an explanation for what was happening. I let it go and kind of forgot about it for a few days, until I happened to put my tongue against my upper gums on the right side. *Huh*, I thought. *There's definitely some swelling going on there. That's weird, I've never had swelling in my gums before; it's really bizarre.*

This time, I decided to try a different route: my dentist. I called my local dentist in Connecticut, who was able to squeeze me in. He examined my mouth and gums and then took a few X-rays. I waited for the results while lying in the patient's chair and checking emails on my phone. I didn't think this was any kind of big deal, until the dentist put the X-rays up on the board across the room and checked them out.

"Hey, Jon, please give me a minute," he said, flicking off the X-ray screen and shooting out of the room.

Uh-oh. This can't be good.

I heard his voice on the phone from his office around the corner. I couldn't tell who he was talking to or what he was saying, but his voice had a concerned tone. My hypochondriac mind went into a tailspin wondering what was going on.

The dentist returned a couple of minutes later, having lost any sign of his usual cheerful demeanor. He took a deep breath, looked me in the eyes, and said, "I want you to go right now to see an oral surgeon in Southport. He's got a full schedule, but he said he would squeeze you in today. I want him to look at your X-rays."

My alarm bells were ringing off the hook. "What is it, doctor? Should I be nervous?"

The dentist refused to commit to anything one way or the other. "Let's just see what the oral surgeon says."

I left the dentist's office and drove straight to the oral surgeon. I was led into an examination room right away and sat down. My X-rays were already up on the wall when the oral surgeon entered and introduced himself. "I'm glad I was able to fit you in, Jon," he said.

"Okay . . . what is it?"

"I can't say just yet," he replied. "But I see why your dentist would send you over here right away. On the surface, this looks like something we might need to be concerned about. But before I can say anything, let's take a CAT scan."

I went into a darkened room, where I was positioned standing in a specific spot and had to remain motionless. A rotating machine did a 360-degree circle around my head. I followed the nurse back to the chair in the examination room. A few minutes later, the oral surgeon returned. He clicked a few times on a computer monitor and angled it in front of me so I could view the screen.

"I'd like you to look at this with me," he stated, gesturing left and right on the images of my face. "See this on the left side of your face? This is what it *should* look like—perfectly normal. Now . . . the *right side* is a different matter. There's something very wrong here. *There is no bone here.* I don't know why."

We were both at a loss. "No bone? What does that mean? How could I not have any bone?"

"Like I said, I don't know why just yet. I would like to do a biopsy *right now*."

Now the shit was getting real. This was all happening so fast. My mind wandered to all kinds of worst-case scenarios . . .

The doctor set up the biopsy, extracting a sample from my gums. It was freaking painful, but it wasn't as if I had any kind of choice. During the process, the oral surgeon said, "I just want to make sure I have enough. We don't want to have to do this again."

After the procedure was completed, the doctor said the sample was going to be rushed off to a lab in Forest Hills, Queens.

"I'll call you as soon as I hear something," he said.

I called Mara the instant I left the oral surgeon's office. I must have sounded panic-stricken—which I was—but she remained calm and reassuring. "Look, we don't know anything yet. Let's not jump to conclusions until we get the results back."

As the days passed, I struggled to get the biopsy out of my mind. Meanwhile, the swelling kept getting worse; I couldn't tell if it was psychological or not. I needed answers, but what I heard next wasn't what I had in mind.

June 19, 2021. I will never forget the exact moment when the oral surgeon called me. I remember standing upstairs in my house, right outside my bedroom doorway. As the conversation began, I kept trying to convince myself it was nothing serious, I was just being my usual neurotic self.

"Jon," he said, "I don't know how to tell you this."

Oh, fuck. Not knowing how to tell a patient something is always a bad fucking sign.

"I'm sorry to say that your biopsy tested positive for lymphoma," he informed me. "I don't have specific details and don't know what kind of lymphoma it is yet . . . but I wanted you to know the result as soon as possible, just so you're aware."

I was so numb and petrified that I ended the conversation without even asking the doctor the obvious question: *What the fuck is lymphoma?*

The first thing I did was play Dr. Google and search *lymphoma*. My worst fears were realized: It's a form of cancer.

Oh God, I have cancer. I'm gonna die. I'm a dead man walking.

I called Mara right away and filled her in. I doubt my voice ever sounded shakier.

Once again, she was an absolute champion and unbelievably steady. "I'm so sorry, Jon . . . this really sucks. Look, the doctor said he doesn't know all the details, right? For now, there isn't anything we can do. We shouldn't assume the worst. We'll know more when we get the full report. Whatever it is, we'll tackle it together, right?"

As always, she'd made me feel somewhat better. "Okay . . ."

Nothing she could say, however, was going to stop this from being scary as fuck. It had gotten real. The area in the sinuses continued to worsen and enlarge. A noticeable bump appeared on my face. I kept thinking the lymphoma was going straight into my nose, my eyes, and my brain.

You'd think things couldn't get any worse, but they did. On June 21—just two days after I received my cancer diagnosis—my mother, Elaine Schwartz, passed away suddenly at seventy-nine years of age. She had Alzheimer's and dementia, but neither was the cause of death. Without getting into details—that's a whole other story—there was some negligence at the assisted living facility where she was staying.

My mother and I had always been close. We had a ton of mutual respect. I inherited all my business acumen from her. She was an amazing single mom to my sister and me as we were growing up. She was super smart, having been a financial planner until she got sick. She loved Mara and playing grandma with our kids, who called her *gramme*.

My life became a total blur. We went to the cemetery in Ossining, New York, for the funeral, as this is where all Westchester Jews are apparently required to get buried. It was a small ceremony, just a few family members. As I looked around at the other family headstones, I noticed that hardly anyone made it past their fifties—my uncles, my aunts, everybody. *During the funeral, I kept thinking, What the fuck is wrong with my family? I got the worst genes imaginable—the Charlie Brown family tree.*

After the ceremony, my uncle asked if we should be donating anything to charity or giving any of my mother's stuff somewhere specific. Out of nowhere, my younger sister, Stefanie, suggested, "Mom would have wanted a lymphoma charity."

"Why that one?" my uncle asked. "I don't know anybody in our family who has lymphoma."

Stefanie shrugged and the conversation faded. This wasn't the best time to share the news of my health crisis.

The next day, I tried to absorb losing my mother while I was going crazy trying to figure out the smartest course of action to deal with the lymphoma.

I have fucking cancer. I should be receiving the best medical care possible. I want the number one hospital, the top doctors, and the most aggressive treatments possible to eliminate this fucking thing.

It hit me: Memorial Sloan Kettering Cancer Center—also known as MSK—in Manhattan. Somehow, I already knew it was the best and became determined to receive all my tests and treatments there.

I contacted my primary doctor and let him know what was happening. He knew an oncologist at the network where he worked and recommended that I give her a try. My better senses told me to go to the top cancer hospital. Little did I realize how difficult it is to "break into" MSK. They have something like a hundred operators answering phones. I tried every pitch possible to get through, explaining that I had lymphoma and desperately needed to get into their system.

Each operator provided the same response: "I'm sorry, sir, there's nothing we can do."

"Why the fuck not? I don't understand what you're talking about. You're a cancer hospital, right? I've been diagnosed with cancer."

"I'm sorry, sir, I can't help you without the full pathology report. We need to have this in the hospital records. We also need the original tissue sample from your biopsy. Then we'll have to retest it."

I entered a really dark place. I was always used to being in control, and suddenly I wasn't. I felt like I was stuck in quicksand.

I'm dying, and there's nothing I can do about it.

I retried the oral surgeon, pushing him as hard as possible to rush the full pathology report. His hands were tied: This takes weeks to complete.

Weeks? Do I even have weeks left to live?

I confided in Stefanie about my predicament. She's a nutritionist, but I went to her as a sounding board for all my medical stuff. She's a year younger than I am, and we were never that close growing up, but things changed as the years passed. I think my mother brought us together more.

My sister was a caretaker like no other. She had helped with my mother's situation, and she became a godsend to me. I told her about my struggles to hook up with a doctor at MSK. An hour after we hung up, she called to let me know about the conversation she just had with Merri, her girlfriend at the time. It turns out that Merri's college roommate happened to be a lymphoma specialist at MSK.

A lymphoma specialist at MSK—what are the fucking odds?

"I've never called in a favor to her," Merri told my sister. "But I'm going to do it right now."

I received a call from this oncology doctor that same evening. I told her about all my frustration getting through to MSK and my desperation to speak to somebody—*anybody*—who could enter me into that hospital.

"Yeah, that's just how it is, that's the process," she said. "But I'll tell you what. Send me the partial pathology report and I'll see what I can do."

I sent the report to her immediately, and she called me back the next day. "Look, I am an oncologist with a specialty in lymphoma. But, if I were you, I would want this other guy. He's the one you really want. I'll set you up, just say the word."

"Wow," I said, unable to contain my emotions. "I can't believe you would do that for me. You're amazing. Thank you so much."

The doctor made an appointment for me with her colleague for that Thursday. I met with the doctor in the flesh for the first time. Right away, he struck me as the real deal. Not only did he have impeccable credentials and the right affiliations, he also looked and acted the part of the King of Lymphoma. He was a handsome guy in his sixties with a wide smile. He knew his shit. He shook my hand, asked a few questions, did a lightning-fast exam, and mumbled a few explanations before saying he'd already checked out my CAT scan and wanted to run a battery of tests ASAP.

Hell, yeah—I'm in.

We went from CAT scan to PET scan to ultrasound to blood work. *Boom boom boom.* This place rocked. Of course, they couldn't do anything until the full results came in from these tests, along with the full pathology on the biopsy.

When all was said and done, the doctor returned to the exam room. His smile had vanished. "Jon," he began in a consoling voice.

This is not good. Definitely not good.

"You have stage four cancer."

There it is. Stage four. How many stages are there? That's gotta be the worst. Four sounds like the last one before they toss your ass in a coffin.

I completely froze. I couldn't blink, much less say a word.

"Listen, this is what it means," he continued.

I was trying hard to pay attention, but reality was phasing in and out. Everything seemed fuzzy and unreal.

"Your body is divided into three sections . . ." he explained.

Three sections? What am I, a fucking triangle?

"You have cancer in all three of them."

Of course I do. On a good day, Major League baseball players go three for three: three hits in three at bats. I go three for three with cancer.

"Listen, I'm going to walk you through a few things. You only noticed the problem in your sinus . . . but you also have tumors in the groin and in the ribs. Right here . . . and over here."

He gestured for me to feel around those specific areas. While I couldn't detect anything by the ribs, I did notice the tumor in the groin.

Holy shit. That was there all along? Fuck!

"Hey, doctor, I have to ask . . . what are the chances of success?"

"There are a lot of considerations, Jon," he said. "Your age, the type of cancer, where it's spread, etcetera. The bad news is that it's stage four. Chemo doesn't always work, but statistically it works better against lymphoma than other types of cancer. I would say it's about a 70% success rate."

That sounded encouraging, although my brain couldn't calculate that in terms of exact batting average in baseball. It sounded like about two hits in three at bats, which would be something like a .667 batting average—that's amazing, right?

Before he could initiate any kind of treatment, however, we still had to wait for the full pathology and the sample. While I waited, I was a total fucking mess. I couldn't eat, I couldn't sleep, I couldn't talk to anyone, I couldn't think straight.

The symptoms continued to progress. My face turned numb. I couldn't feel my lips or tongue. My gums completely swelled up. The lump in my sinus had blown up to the size of a golf ball.

I didn't want to alarm my kids, but I couldn't hide my terror and misery. I'll never forget the look of concern in my daughter's eyes. It felt devastating.

A couple more days passed when I received a call from the doctor. "The full pathology results are in, Jon, and have been thoroughly reviewed. My staff and I discussed your situation and agree we need to be aggressive with your treatment. Pack your bags and come in. You're starting chemotherapy *today*."

Mara and I didn't waste a split second. I wanted that treatment so fucking badly. I knew it was the only way I was going to survive. We tossed some random things into a bag and sped off to MSK.

I was checked into the hospital on arrival. I put on the gown, after which an army of nurses and practitioners barraged me with questions as they stuffed a thermometer in my mouth, harpooned an IV needle into my arm, tested my blood pressure, and so on. One of the on-call doctors asked how I was doing.

"Oh, great, it's like the Carlton Hotel in Cannes," I remarked.

"Good—I'm glad you have a sense of humor—it helps," he chuckled.

They set me up with what they call an R-CHOP panel, which includes five drugs known to combat non-Hodgkin lymphoma. I did four rounds of punishing cocktails once every three weeks. My hair fell out. I puked my guts out. I hated every second, but worked my way through it, largely thanks to Mara being a rock by my side and the thought that at some point this would all be over.

The thing about chemo is that it's poison. It kills fucking everything: the bad stuff, the good stuff, and everything in between. The smell flooded my entire body: my pores, my skin, my nose, my head, my chest. Then I flushed it out with constant liquids and peeing. The cycle is absolute hell.

R-CHOP was only the first half. Once that finished, I had to go through a few weeks of what they call the R-ICE cocktail, which is an acronym for three drugs with idiotic-sounding names you don't need to know about. The doctors compared my body to a lawn that had just been perfectly manicured with R-CHOP. There are no visible weeds, but underneath there could be all kinds of bad shit brewing. The R-ICE targets everything below the surface that the tests don't reveal. Cancer cells are pesky sons of bitches; they can be microscopic and hide so well that the tests fail to detect them.

Six months elapsed from when I was first diagnosed with lymphoma. I went through another round of tests—including a PET scan—and steeled myself for the worst. The doctor's wide smile had returned—a good sign. "Jon—I'm pleased to say that your results came in clean. As of right now, you are *cancer-free.*"

That's right, cancer, I beat you! You can go fuck yourself...

Chapter One

I Lived Off Stouffer's French Bread Pizza

WORK ASIDE, WE COME TO NEW YORK FOR THE POSSIBILITY OF INTERACTION AND INSPIRATION.
—DAVID BYRNE

I don't think anyone is going to give a shit about most of my early life, so to avoid boring you to tears, I'm going to cover the highlights and rush through the rest.

I was born in New Rochelle, New York, on October 3, 1966. My parents lived in Riverdale at the time and then moved to Hartsdale. I don't remember much about our time in Hartsdale, except when I was about five a dog nearly bit my ear off. For some reason, I didn't hold a grudge against dogs and continue to love them to this day.

We settled in Chappaqua when I was in second grade. We lived in a modest, three-bedroom Cape with a little brook in the backyard. The place desperately needed remodeling and decorating—my mom didn't mind old floral wallpaper—but none of that was a priority at the time.

My early claim to fame was that I set the school record for what I believe was called the shuttle run. The kids would be led to a basketball court, where we'd run to a line, pick up a block, and drop it off. We'd do the same thing at a second, third, and fourth line. Olympic-level stuff, right? I don't know what possessed me that day, but I was lightning. My record held for many years, but I'm certain that it's since been shattered. That was the full extent of my athletic career.

Like every other kid, I dreamed of being a star baseball player and hitting a game-winning homerun. I loved baseball—especially the New York Mets—and went to games at Shea Stadium with my friends as often as I could. The Mets were a lousy team in the late 1970s—especially after they traded away their ace, legendary pitcher Tom Seaver—but they had six-foot-six Dave Kingman, who hit 500-foot homeruns and mile-high popups that never came down. Mostly, though, he struck out five times a game.

I have so many great memories of going to Shea in those days. They lost a good chunk of the time, of course, but the upper deck tickets were only about five bucks, and the stadium always had fun things going on. They were ahead of their time with fan banner days and promotional giveaways, like expensive coolers and cups, which were way more valuable than the tickets.

My friend Keith was my Mets wingman, but I probably picked up my love for the team from my dad, Herb Schwartz. Outside of that and my future career path—which I'll get to—I don't have many good things to say about my father. My mom, Elaine, divorced him when I was around ten because he was a serial cheater. He became something of a weekend dad, but he was a deadbeat when it came to child support and helping my mother, my sister, Stefanie, and me. Mom was left to do everything singlehandedly, such as getting us to school, making sure we did our homework, and filling the refrigerator. I lived off Stouffer's French Bread Pizza, which was fine by me; it was (and is) delicious. Mom also organized my Bar Mitzvah, which was a fun event, although I was at my absolute worst at that time: ugly gold-framed glasses, shiny steel braces, and a thirteen-year-old voice that cracked like a wounded animal.

As I mentioned in the Introduction, mom granted Stefanie and me a lot of freedom—right up until I got in trouble, which only happened once when my friends and I were arrested for stealing a stretchy eraser from a five and dime store. My mom came down to the store and had to bail us out. She was pissed. I learned a valuable lesson and realized I'd screwed up a good thing. I never did anything like that again and had to work hard to earn back her trust.

I was 100 percent on team Elaine (mom), but that isn't to say that I don't have a few fond memories with my dad. He'd take us to see cool movies and go slot car racing. I enjoyed staying in his apartment in New York because we'd have amazing pizza, and I'd get exposure to the sprawling city that I'd come to love.

He also had a ton of cable TV channels we didn't have at our house in Chappaqua. The best of these was the notoriously explicit Channel J, which featured an eyeful of porn that was essential viewing for the development of a preteen male in the late-1970s and early 80s. I couldn't believe all the nude action I was seeing with my virgin eyes: Robin Byrd, large-breasted porn stars, hot Asian women under waterfalls . . . those were the days! My underage imagination kept plotting how I might hook up with the women whose phone numbers flitted across the screen, but the logistics of being in my dad's apartment—not to mention that I had no money and was way underage—always seemed to get in the way. It goes without saying my dad disapproved of my flipping to these channels, but once I found out about them, there was no stopping me.

For all his flaws, my dad built a respectable career in . . . drum roll . . . sales and commercial production. It runs in the family, I suppose. At one time, my dad represented some of the biggest commercial directors in the business and made enough money to move out to Beverly Hills. He was also the king of bad decision-making. He overspent, gambled, remarried, and had three more kids—my half-siblings. This second marriage was doomed as well, ending in divorce. Eventually, he went bankrupt.

I don't regret having grown up in Chappaqua and, in fact, there was one major benefit to having attended high school in the mid-1980s: The football Giants used to train at nearby Pace University. This meant they frequented the same bars I did—Michael's and Foley's. I saw players nearly every night, especially legendary linebacker LT (Lawrence Taylor), who didn't pay much attention to team curfews. Once a week, Michael's had a comedy night, and you never knew what chaos LT might cause. Often, he would pull up a chair in front of the comedian's microphone, sit in it, cross his arms, and bark, "Make me laugh!" Brutal for the stand-ups, but hilarious for everyone else.

I never fit in with the preppies and stuck-up girls in junior high and high school. But I managed to find my core group of best friends: Jeff, Ed, and Keith. We shared a love of sports, music, and girls and went to many baseball games and concerts in the city together. As I've said, I was a punk rock kid who was immersed in the Ramones, the Clash, the Sex Pistols, the Pogues, Social Distortion, Hūsker Dū, Pixies, Devo, Violent Femmes, Buzzcocks, Descendents, the Replacements . . . you get the idea. I had all their albums and played them to death. My world was built around music, and to this day, I can't believe how lucky I was to have seen several of my favorite bands live on stage when they were in their prime.

I was fortunate in another respect. Although my friends and I were considered outsiders in our own school, we did well with the girls at the high school on the less fancy side of town. They were just more accessible and approachable. Suddenly, I was able to date a lot of girls and, as it was described back then, get some action.

When I was about fifteen, my girlfriend and I started fooling around on the shag rug of her parents' living room floor, thinking the house was going to be empty for a while. It wasn't. I was mid-thrust when her father came barreling into the room and chased me around the house. I barely had time to grab my clothes and fly out of there buck naked. If he'd had a shotgun, I would have been a goner.

"Don't you ever see my daughter or come back here again!" he threatened.

That's what I call a rough ending to a relationship.

Flash forward a few years: Somehow, I made it through high school and was accepted into SUNY Plattsburgh, which is about a half hour from the Canadian border. There were two commercials in Montreal that were piped on our local cable stations: Bar B Barn Ribs—which was a mediocre Dallas barbecue like you might find in New York City—and Club Super Sexe, which was a strip club like no other. My friends and I were in heaven spending our weekends going back and forth across the border to frequent these joints. Occasionally, we'd catch a Montreal Expos game during the day; the stadium was always empty, and the bleacher seats were even cheaper than at Shea—around a Canadian dollar. For the return trip, we were allowed to take back one case of beer per person. Molson Brador, of course.

Plattsburgh had its share of thrills, too. My friends and I would frequent the local redneck bars. There was also a local Air Force base nearby, so there was always a lot of friction between the local guys and the military. Several of my friends were on the rugby team or played hockey, so they were tough and welcomed bar fights. On the other hand, I was a skinny, wimpy kid who got my ass kicked a bunch of times in those bars. On one occasion we got into a brawl reminiscent of the movie *Roadhouse*; fists, chairs, and tables were flying. I made my way behind the bar with a pool stick and managed to whack a goliath who was coming at me in the head, knocking him out.

Then there were the Plattsburgh college girls. Holy shit, they were crazy and wild. The girls from the other side of the tracks in Chappaqua had nothing on them. I was a kid in a candy store, spending every night with a different girl. In my mind, I was making up for lost time.

Oh yeah, I also took classes in college and majored in Business Marketing, although I barely remember any of it. Obviously, it wasn't that challenging, as I was able to graduate in 1988 with around a 3.0 average without having put in much effort.

My first job out of college was working as a peon at J.P. Morgan in New York City. I don't even remember my job title there. Whatever it was, I couldn't stand it. I spent my whole day inputting information into a database. I'm sure I wasn't very good at it and had a bad attitude. My manager hated me. The best thing about my two years working there was the free all-you-can-eat lunch.

There were upsides, of course. I was young, earning a steady paycheck, and living in the city with a couple of my close friends, who also had crappy starter jobs. We shared a two-bedroom on the border of Spanish Harlem and, with our low salaries and high expenses, barely scraped by. A big night out on the town was going to nickel beer nights at bars.

My next couple of jobs were so shitty I don't even remember them. I think I was selling investments for an insurance company or something like that. I felt like I was going nowhere and desperately needed to do something I was passionate about.

I started to become curious about what my dad was doing at a production company, representing directors. It seemed way more interesting than my job, and I always liked sales. To my father's credit, he gave me a few industry contacts. I emailed them all and heard nothing back for a while. Months later, I received a reply out of the blue. I became an assistant sales rep for the whopping salary of $18,000 a year. Essentially, the job involved dialing for dollars. Over time, I became good at it—who knew? Within three or so years, I built a Rolodex of nearly 150 contacts. Suddenly, I was contributing and of value to somebody.

This job led to my working for Jeff Feuerzeig, a talented documentary director (whose best-known film, *The Devil and Daniel Johnston*, would eventually earn him the Documentary Directing Award at the Sundance Festival in 2005). I learned a lot from Jeff, and he was extremely supportive of me, helping build up my career.

Jeff perhaps did one of the most pivotal things that ever happened to me: introducing me to Joshua Blum, who founded an independent production and management company called Washington Square Films in 1995. At the time, WSF was best known for its five-part PBS series, *United States of Poetry*.

In June 1997, Josh agreed to meet me for coffee. He came across as such a mellow, easygoing guy—not at all what I expected. We talked as if we'd known each other for years. My intuition was telling me this was a business match made in heaven; he was laid-back while I was a bit more brash and opinionated. I felt I could work well with him and said to myself that I couldn't afford to fuck this up.

I laid all my cards on the table, telling him I would do anything it takes to be successful; I just needed to find the right home.

"What do you think about getting into the commercial side of the business?" I asked.

"I don't know much about commercials," Josh admitted.

"Don't worry about it," I said. "Jeff and I will teach you all there is to know."

"Great," he concluded. "Jeff likes you, and I already trust you. Let's give it a shot. I'll let you do your thing."

We shook hands: I landed the job at WSF. I knew there would be a lot of upside. I became determined to make this work.

I dove in headfirst, showing up at the WSF office at 9 a.m.—days before I was supposed to start.

"What are you doing here?" Josh asked.

"I thought I would start today," I sheepishly answered.

It was an inauspicious beginning, but at least I impressed him with my eagerness. I was all in with my new job and anxious to make my mark. But then I became involved in something that nearly blew everything up before it had a chance to get started . . .

Chapter Two

May the Schwartzes Be with Us

> MARRIAGE IS WORSE THAN DYING. WHY STAY WITH ONE PERSON FOR FIFTY YEARS? WE ADVISE AGAINST MARRIAGE.
> —JOEY RAMONE

I should state for the record that I *strongly disagree* with the Joey Ramone quote above, which I've included only for comic relief. (This disclaimer may or may not be because my wife was looking over my shoulder as I was writing this and shouted, "Hey, Jon—*what the fuck*?!")

Let's backtrack a bit to 1990 before returning to work stuff and my cliffhanger. At the time, I was living with my best friend Jeff in an apartment on the Upper West Side across from the Beacon Theatre. We went on a lot of double dates together, so it wasn't unusual when a girl he was seeing from the University of Albany brought along a college friend for me.

Her name was Mara, and she was obviously still in college, whereas I had already graduated and was working in some shitty job that I hated. I wouldn't say it was "love at first sight" or anything corny like that, but *man*, was I attracted to her. She had kinky, multicolored hair—mostly, dyed red and brown—and an *incredible* body. To my surprise, Mara has just given me clearance to write that I was mesmerized by her *really nice boobs*. Hey, I'm a guy—it's an honest answer.

Anyway, while Mara and I were in the apartment getting to know each other—during which time she told me she was originally from Long Island—Jeff and his date slipped away to our tiny one bedroom, where the couple made no effort to conceal that they were—well, doing more than talking. I wouldn't have been surprised if the audience at the Beacon Theatre across the street heard it, too, and gave them a standing ovation. Mara and I laughed things off as best we could.

During a brief pause in our conversation, I pulled the smooth move of asking Mara to lie down with me on the couch. She gave that a hard pass. As I recall, her exact words were, "Not gonna happen!" Fortunately, I came across as more of a likeable dope than a pushy jerk, so I was able to turn things around. We hit it off well enough for her to agree to see me again for a real date with just the two of us. We met a couple of days later and ended up walking around the Lincoln Center area. It felt natural and we had a ton of laughs. Neither of us was looking for a serious relationship at the time, but the whole time I kept thinking: There's something here . . .

I definitely wanted to see her again. And again. And again. It became tricky because she was still at Albany, and I had to schlep all the way up there to see her. (Not that it wasn't worth it.) Our dates were always on the cheap because of my shit salary, but she didn't seem to mind because we had so many great times together.

A few months passed and I was totally hooked—so much, in fact, that I left her a handwritten note in her Albany apartment telling her I loved her. Pretty romantic, right?

She read it to herself and became deathly silent. Then she grunted the two words a guy does not want to hear after having said *I love you* to his girlfriend: "Thank you."

Uh-oh. Absolute, utter failure. Houston, we have a problem.

I felt like a schmuck and thought I'd blown the whole thing. To this day, I'm still rattled by her reaction. I don't know how I recovered from it. I guess I was more resilient than I thought, because I sucked it up and tried again—in person—a few days later.

This time, to my relief, she said, "I love you, too."

A miracle! I'd won her over.

After we married on Long Island in 1994, we lived in the city for a while and eventually searched for a town where we could plant roots. I told her I would never live on Long Island and wanted a change of pace from Westchester. We concentrated our search in southern Connecticut and went up and down the coast and looked at every town. We couldn't afford Greenwich. The schools were bad in Stamford. And Darien had no Jews.

We finally found the perfect suburban town in Fairfield, where we bought a beautiful house. Fairfield, located along what is known as "the Gold Coast," borders Westport, Trumbull, Easton, Bridgeport, and Weston. It has some beautiful little beaches, lots of trees, two colleges (Sacred Heart and Fairfield University), a decent-sized Jewish community, and good public schools. It's perhaps best known for being the home of Frank Pepe Pizzeria Napoletana (not the more famous one in New Haven) and Super Duper Weenie hot dog restaurant. In the years we've called Fairfield home, the town has come a long way with some fantastic metropolitan-caliber restaurants and entertainment venues. Fairfield was also attractive because it was commutable by Metro-North into the city, where I figured I'd always be working.

About a year after our move, we were ready to have kids. We tried for several months but nothing happened. We went for all kinds of tests, but they couldn't pinpoint a specific reason for why Mara couldn't get pregnant. We tried intrauterine insemination (IUI) three times without success. We next moved on to in vitro fertilization (IVF), where we faced a complication—but not the one you might think.

I know I'm probably going to oversimplify IVF or explain it completely wrong, but during the process, they take out Mara's eggs, mix them up with my boys, and then implant the three best of the lot. We were told there was a chance we might have triplets—which we absolutely did not want—but went with it anyway. The day they were supposed to be fertilized was written in stone; any deviation from this date meant failure.

As fate would have it, the worst snowstorm of the decade hit Connecticut the day of our appointment. All the highways and roads were shut down. But we had no choice. We had to somehow get from our house in Fairfield to the Norwalk medical facility during a total whiteout. We miraculously made it on to highway 95, where there wasn't a single other vehicle in sight (or a road, for that matter). We hydroplaned the whole way there.

Miraculously, we made it to the fertility clinic—and so did the doctor. He did the entire procedure himself, as no one else on his staff was able to make it in through the storm.

A few weeks later, the doctor informed us that IVF was a success. In fact, we were having twins. We were so happy after having gone through all those hoops to get to that point.

That turned out to be just the first step in a long road of trials and tribulations. We went in for a routine sixteen-week checkup and thought everything was going great; Mara wasn't having any issues. During the examination, the doctor informed us that her cervix was deteriorating. Mara needed surgery the next day. We were told she would be on bedrest the rest of the pregnancy. The procedure was supposed to be quick—maybe an hour at most. After an excruciating three hours, the doctor came out and described to me how membranes were hanging out, putting the twins at grave risk. They sent Mara straight to the emergency room. For the rest of the term—about four months—she had to remain in the maternity ward, basically lying with her head upside down. They put a terbutaline pump in her leg to stop contractions. I couldn't even imagine what it felt like for her with the blood rushing to her head 24/7. I know she was incredibly uncomfortable and suffered massive headaches. It was challenging enough for her to be able to think, but then they gave her a massive amount of magnesium, which caused severe (though temporary) memory loss.

While Mara was on strict bedrest in the maternity ward, I was commuting back and forth from Fairfield to New York City for work and then driving to visit her in Stamford. I did this every day for four months, rinse and repeat. It was a tense, hellish time for both of us, but obviously a ton worse for her than me.

Finally, on September 1, 2001, the twins—Alissa and Matthew (Matt)—entered the world. They were premature and under-developed, as expected—but at least they were born. For Mara, it couldn't have been a greater relief.

Alissa's birth was okay; she came out crying and the medical team did their usual stuff for preemies. She stayed in the hospital for about ten days with a special lamp for a touch of jaundice, but was otherwise fine.

When Matt was born, however, we heard nothing—not a peep. We knew this couldn't have been good. They whisked him away, saying, "Don't worry, you'll see him later." They didn't give us a clue what was wrong.

"Later" turned out to be several days, as the medical team struggled to keep Matt alive. He wasn't breathing on his own, so they put a tube in him and pumped him with antibiotics. For a while, the doctors didn't think he was going to make it, as he wasn't showing enough improvement. A month or so went by. Just at the point that we thought it was "game over," Matt's body at last began to accept the medications and he started to breathe on his own.

On September 11, 2001, while Alissa was under three pounds, we were told she was in good enough shape to take home. That morning, as we sped down highway 95 to pick her up, we heard reports on the radio about the attacks on the World Trade Center. The first plane hit . . . and then another one. On what should have been one of the happiest days of our lives, the world was collapsing. Everything shut down.

The hospital was buzzing when we arrived there. The attacks were all everybody talked about. All the televisions around the hospitals showed the horrific news footage. Patients, visitors, and medical staff were constantly on their phones checking on status of people they knew. The heliport was activated because they thought there might be patient spillover from the city hospitals. Rooms and equipment were readied for the worst. But no injured people ever showed. There were no survivors from the collapse of the Twin Towers.

Mara and I experienced such a crazy mix of emotions. We were supposed to be happy that our child was finally coming home with us. But there was no way we could celebrate with all this tragedy going on.

Somehow, with the help of family members, we made it through the early days with two needy twins during this unbelievable time in history. Mara was bedridden for so long that she had to relearn how to walk. She had contracted an infection—possibly what had been passed through to Matt and caused all his trauma—and was on all kinds of medications. In the middle of all this, she had to figure out how to breastfeed two premature twins who needed to gain weight fast.

Matt and Alissa were constantly in and out of doctors' appointments. When they are that little, anything can go wrong, and we had to pull out all the stops to help them grow bigger and stronger.

Matt was especially fussy and challenging. He just wouldn't sleep. The only way we could get him down was to drive around for a while and park at the beach until he'd fall asleep. It took us a year and half to figure out that his body couldn't handle dairy.

Other problems surfaced. He was diagnosed with asthma, which meant he needed regular chest X-rays. One round of tests revealed that he had a diaphragmatic hernia, which required immediate surgery. We found the best pediatric surgeon at Yale to put everything in place. A three-hour surgery turned out to be six. It was touch and go there for a while.

It's a massive understatement to say that Matt had a rough early childhood. Somehow, we all came through it all as a stronger family, which would prove to be an invaluable asset for us years later. But that part of my story comes much later . . . now it's time to return to a comical part of my life story, which happened to be timed with the start of my career.

Chapter Three

My Beef with Bryan Adams

> I THINK ANGER IS AN UNDERUSED EMOTION.
> —JOHN LYDON

As I've mentioned, I am not a musician—I don't play any instrument, not even air guitar—or an athlete. However, I *am* a serious collector and have been doing it for years. I own a ton of valuable stuff capturing classic moments in music and sports that have been signed by some all-time greats. I would go to all kinds of weird events to meet these superstars, including conventions, department stores, sneaker stores, and record stores (when they existed, that is).

My goal was always to try to get something visually interesting for the legendary musician or athlete to sign. In one instance, I was able to combine my two passions in one and get all the Ramones to sign a baseball bat. Why on earth I had them sign a baseball bat is anyone's guess; maybe I had been inspired by their song "Beat on the Brat." This was tricky because the

Ramones were a rotating cast, and by this time, they all hated each other. Bassist Dee Dee Ramone was probably the toughest to obtain, because he was suffering from anorexia, bulimia, and depression and had quit the band after the *Brain Drain* album to become a rapper under the name Dee Dee King.

By late 1997, my white electric guitar featured at least a dozen legendary signatures in blue Sharpie marker on the front and back. I was always precise with my instructions to everyone who signed it: "Use this blue Sharpie and only sign your name. Please, don't personalize it in any way by writing 'To Jonathan' or 'Dear Jonathan.'"

I had good reasons why I was so strict. First, if people had scribbled "To Jonathan" on the guitar, it would have taken up way too much space on the instrument. Second, as a collectible, it would have far less value with personalization (not that I had any intention of selling it). Third, it looked beautiful with just the signatures.

No guitarist ever had a problem with this. Until . . . singer/guitarist Bryan Adams.

Bryan Adams was known for his 1980s hits—"Cuts Like a Knife," "Straight from the Heart," "Summer of 69," and so forth—and was still considered a hot musician well into the following decade. In 1997, he recorded his *Unplugged* album on MTV, which was released on CD not long after that.

At the time, I frequently checked The Village Voice magazine to find out which artists were in the city doing signings. While turning the pages, I spotted a notice that Bryan Adams was going to appear at Sam Goody record store on 51st Street and Sixth Avenue to promote his *Unplugged* CD.

I admit that I wasn't a fan of Bryan Adams at all. I knew he was popular and had some hits. I also considered him the least talented name to appear on my guitar. In my mind, at best he was borderline. I shrugged, thinking, Okay, I have a little room on the guitar. He'll be in the city, and I have the time, so it's easy. What the fuck, I'm just gonna' do it.

I went to Sam Goody, bought the CD, and had it in my hand with my priceless guitar. The line strung around the block, but once I was there with the guitar, invested in the purchase, and waiting, there was no turning back.

The crowd inched forward. An hour or so later, I finally made it to the front. Bryan was behind the table with an unknown session musician. I gathered that the two had performed something of a mini concert in the store before the signing.

I put the CD down on the table and held the guitar upright with my Sharpie. "Hi, Bryan, nice to meet you," I began in a polite tone. "Look, I have a huge favor. You can see there are a lot of other famous guitarist signatures on here. I'd just like you to sign your name on it without personalizing it."

Bryan took the guitar and his own Sharpie. I can't explain why, but the air became thick with tension. I could feel something was about to go terribly wrong.

"What's your name?" he asked.

"It's Jonathan," I replied. "But—please don't write my name on there. Just sign your name in that blank spot over there."

While I knew he heard me, I could tell he just didn't give a shit. I saw problems all over this. "Oh God, here we go," I huffed under my breath.

I could tell he was scribbling a lot more than he should have. My blood started to boil. I was about to reach for the guitar when he presented it to the session musician. "Hey, sign this," Bryan ordered. "He wants your autograph on it, too."

The guy looked at me and could tell from my expression that this was a bad idea. He hesitated, not wanting to do it. His eyes indicated "Leave me out of this."

"Go on, sign the side—there's plenty of room there," Bryan egged him on. "Address it 'To Jonathan.'"

The session musician shrugged as if to say to me, "Sorry, he's the boss." He opened the Sharpie and signed the side of the guitar.

No offense to the session musician, but I didn't know who he was and certainly didn't want his name anywhere on this guitar alongside those legends. This was turning into a blizzard of a shitstorm.

I can't speak for what was on Bryan's mind or explain why he did this. He struck me as a cold guy, maybe a bit brash. To him, this was all business. Whatever the case, he was obviously interested in personalizing everything. Maybe he didn't want to sign something only to have it sold online; it was the early days of eBay and celebrities were starting to get cautious.

The session musician handed the guitar back to me. He and Bryan had both personalized their signatures with the words "To Jonathan."

It was fucking ruined. The more I looked it, the more I seethed with rage. There is no other way to describe my actions, except to say that I completely lost my shit.

"Why do you have to be such an asshole?!" I shouted at Bryan.

He waved me off like a king to a peasant. "Oh, come on—I signed your guitar. What's your problem?"

"You personalized my guitar. I specifically told you not to do that!" I raged.

"Yeah, yeah," Bryan sighed. "What are you going to do about it?"

His taunting infuriated me even further. I turned beet red and began to sweat profusely. My body shook. People crowded in closer to get a better look at what was happening. The shit was going down. I could sense everything was closing in around me.

I grabbed his buttoned-down shirt with both hands. He wasn't the kind of guy who backed down from a fight. He latched onto my hoodie. I curled my fist, preparing to take a swing and knock him on his ass.

Before my knuckles could land on his jaw, a large security guy threw me to the floor. I was hauled across the store and tossed out the front door like a bag of trash. Somehow, I'd managed to hold on to the guitar and CD. I was completely rattled, covered with sweat, and shaking like I was in another world. Part of me wanted to charge back into the store and tackle Bryan, but common sense took over. I knew I would land right back in this spot, if not end up in jail. So, I picked up my sorry butt and did the walk of shame home.

I stewed about the incident all evening. I tossed and turned all night. I didn't think this was over—not by a longshot. That fucker had ruined my guitar on purpose. I had to do something about it.

I had heard that Bryan Adams was scheduled to appear live the following morning on *The Howard Stern Show* on WXRK-FM radio. As it happens, I was a huge Howard Stern fan and listened to him every morning. I went to work super early and dialed into his show in the hope of stating my case on the air and getting Howard to take my side. The phone rang for a while until Stuttering John, Howard's call screener, answered. My head was spinning as I raced through details of my conflict with Bryan Adams. Stuttering John sounded interested in what I had to say and asked for my number. He ended by saying I should stay close to the phone, as he would be calling me back in about ten minutes.

Sure enough, my phone rang ten minutes later. Stuttering John told me to stay on; I was going to be on the air any second. I heard Howard Stern bantering with Bryan Adams when the subject veered. "Hey, Bryan," Howard said in his inimitable voice, "There's a guy on the phone who says he got into an altercation with you at a record store last night."

"Oh God," Bryan murmured.

Here we go. This is my chance. I don't have much time. I better make it good.

"Hi, Howard, thanks for having me on," I began, trying to sound normal and calm but knowing I didn't. "Last night, I went to Bryan's signing at Sam Goody. I bought the CD and waited on the line for hours. I'd brought my prized electric guitar with me. It has signatures of all these rock gods—Keith Richards, Ray Davies, Robbie Robertson, and so on. I handed the guitar to Bryan and gave explicit instructions: Just sign your name, don't personalize it. So, Bryan takes the guitar and writes 'To Jonathan' on it with a Sharpie. If that's not enough, he orders his session guy to sign the side the same way. I didn't want the guy's autograph or anything on the side. Bryan knew what he was doing. I don't know why he had to be such an asshole."

Howard tried to sound impartial, but I guess he felt he had to hear both sides of the story and be supportive of his guests. "What was this all about, Bryan? This guy still sounds pissed."

"Listen, Howard, you know how it is," Bryan said. "You can't please these autograph collectors all the time. They're always complaining about stuff."

"Yeah, I hear you," Howard followed. "Some of these collectors can sometimes be pains in the asses."

At this point, there was a lot of back-and-forth and overlapping of voices. Not only wasn't I getting any kind of satisfaction; it was becoming a bit of a shit-on-me type situation. I could tell that the guest mikes were always better amplified than the voices of the people who called in, so I had to shout louder to get my point across. This was exactly the kind of entertainment and conflict fans of Howard's show loved. I never thought I'd be involved in one of these situations myself.

"You ruined my guitar!" I insisted. "Why did you have to be such a dick?! All you needed to do was sign your name!"

"You got what you wanted," Bryan flung back. "I didn't do anything wrong."

"I've been collecting autographs on this guitar for years! You have no idea how valuable it is! Why do you have to be such an asshole?!"

"You collectors are all the same, chasing me down," he fired back. "You want this, you want that—you're never satisfied. I'm sick of it."

It went back and forth like that for a while until Bryan got the last word in, and I was cut off. I hung up with mixed feelings. I felt some level of satisfaction that I had challenged Bryan on a popular show. I had released some of my hatred out of my system, which was a bit of a relief. Unfortunately, Bryan hadn't conceded anything, and certainly didn't apologize. I'd like to think that, at the least, I spooked him enough to avoid doing future signings for a while.

Something unexpected happened after I hung up. My phone blew up, as if I had become somebody famous. My dad called. My friends called. Other family members called. I was getting messages from people all over the place from my past. I had no idea how many people I knew listened to *The Howard Stern Show*.

Word spread fast. My coworkers hovered around me like I was the world's biggest celebrity. Total insanity.

I guess I hadn't thought through the possibility that I was going to receive so much notoriety and that it might impact things at work. I'd only been at WSF for a few months, and I'd caused all this commotion. It dawned on me that Josh preferred to keep a low profile. I worried about what he might have been thinking—probably something along the lines of "Who the hell did I just hire?"

Josh had a look of concern when he entered the office. He asked me what happened, so I filled him in on the entire saga. This time, of course, I was a lot less animated. By the end of the story, he kind of just shrugged it off and smiled.

After that incident, I knew I had a lot to prove to Josh—and to myself. I became more determined than ever to make this new commercial division a success.

There was still the matter of my damaged guitar. I couldn't live another second with that son of a bitch's name tarnishing my guitar. I went to a drugstore and bought a bottle of Goo Gone, a product that I hoped would remove the Sharpie. I delicately wiped over and over until the personalization disappeared over time. The affected areas had lost some shine, but overall, Goo Gone did the trick.

Bryan Adams: gone.

Chapter Four

Apple Shoots During the Recession

WHEN I SEE EVERYONE DOING THE SAME THING, I WANT TO DO THE OPPOSITE.
—MIKE NESS

Washington Square Films is unique in that we are more diversified than most companies we are up against, which may explain why we've had such staying power. Josh oversees the whole company—film, television, theater, and management—while I handle the commercial and content production division.

Fortunately, my career didn't come to a screeching halt before it had a chance to start because of the Bryan Adams incident in 1997. Josh hardly knew me at that time and, as I learned right away, he preferred to keep a low profile. "I'm so sorry, Josh," I apologized. "It was such a crazy night. I promise, nothing like that is ever going to happen again."

Like I said, I was determined to make my mark at WSF and show Josh—and everyone else—what I could do. My being part of the small team there somehow felt right, although I was basically starting from scratch. Over time, I earned Josh's trust and proved my value. My full title at WSF became Director of Sales and Marketing and Managing Director, which sounds way more important than it really is. Unless you happen to be in my business, you probably don't have a clue what the title means. When I'm asked, I always answer, "I'm a sales guy."

Some people—especially in my industry—cringe at the word sales. They think it's beneath them or something, like I'm comparing what I do to selling used cars or life insurance. Not for me. I think sales is all about building relationships with people and earning their trust, so they want to work with my company again.

I look at it this way: It's my job to put the puzzle pieces together and try to find the right projects (directing commercials and content) for my directors. These people are super talented, so I work with my sales team and reps from all over the country to keep them as busy as possible working on television commercials and online content. Once we are contacted by an advertising agency or the client, we choose a suitable director from our bench—someone we believe would be a good fit for the project—and submit samples of their work. If they are interested in us, we set up a conference call and send in our bid, along with a comprehensive treatment. Once we've made our presentation, it's in God's hands, as they say. If we are awarded the job, the agreement is set in motion, and everything gets turned over to our production team. I take a backseat to Partner/EP Han West, who does all the heavy lifting.

In conjunction with the director, Han finds the right location, recruits a producer and their team, brings in a casting director, hires a cast, and so much more. Sometimes Han will fire a question my way—"Should we shoot this in Miami or Austin?" or "Do you know of a good producer in Minneapolis?"—but he's the quarterback calling the plays.

Whenever possible, I always try to be on set for the shoot, although I don't have an active role. The line producer is in charge, interfacing with the agency and client. I don't butt in, as I trust the process is in good hands. I'm there because I have the relationships with the clients and it's important that they feel cared for. I'm shmoozing, taking them out for lunch, drinks, or dinner, and listening closely to everything they say. Paying attention is 99% of what I do. I'm thinking, How can I make my client happy? Are there any problems I can solve, even if they haven't specifically asked me?

***

The WSF commercial division started out with one talented documentary film maker and then another, and then we brought on Mark Pellington, who later earned recognition for having directed such notable films as *Arlington Road* and *The Mothman Prophecies*. Earlier, he had worked with Josh on *The United States of Poetry*.

Over the next several years, the WSF commercial business grew by leaps and bounds, and we added several other talented directors to our roster. We entered the business at just the right time. We worked with some top-level clients like Verizon on many of their early spots for their legendary "Can you hear me now?" campaign.

We did a project for a new product launch with Proctor & Gamble in 1999 that was shrouded in secrecy and called something like Project X. After the project was awarded, we went to the agency to meet the creative team and hear the big reveal about the product. The creative director plopped this never-before-seen object on the table. I remember looking at my team and thinking that it looked like a paper towel on a stick. I couldn't imagine who would buy this. God, were we wrong! It went on to sell something like fifty million units. You may have already figured out that the product we had second-guessed was none other than the Swiffer Sweeper.

Every now and then, we did commercials with professional athletes. Hall of Fame NFL quarterback Dan Marino was an amazing guy. He went out of his way to talk to people. He'd go to the crew guys in the corner, put his arm around each person, and ask, "Hey, what do you do?"

Tennis legend Billie Jean King was like that, too. She seemed genuinely curious and asked everyone their names and what they did.

Hall of Fame NFL quarterback and announcer Terry Bradshaw was a pisser. He was so fucking entertaining. We once shot a commercial on his massive estate. After the shoot, he brought out unending kegs of beer for everyone. Instead of hanging out in his house, he spent the entire day hanging out with the agency and client telling joke after joke and cracking us up.

Other celebs hated being on commercial sets, even when they were getting paid upward of $1 million or more for an eight-hour day. I won't name them—you never know when I might need to work with them again. At least there is never a dull moment in my business.

***

One day, Pete—one of our documentary filmmakers—suggested, "Hey, Jon—you know, wouldn't it be great if we could do something with Apple? I mean, they're the hottest company in the world."

Most people might have shrugged it off as a crazy suggestion, thinking it would never happen. But I took it as a challenge.

I went online and searched for as many marketing people at Apple as I could find. I tracked down a bunch of people and shot them cold emails, essentially pitching that they consider working with us and our director. A year went by with no response. The trail went cold.

Out of the blue, long after I'd written off the possibility of getting any kind of response from Apple, I received a phone call from someone in their marketing department. "Hey, Jonathan," she began, "I remember that email you sent me a while back. Look, we're building the 59th Street Apple cube store near FAO Schwarz. We need a little video capturing all the excitement of the opening—people sleeping out the night before, the lines forming, people charging in, etcetera. This is going to be a massive launch."

We eagerly took on the gig. In my mind, it felt like a test to see what we could do and could lead to a ton of other things.

I only saw Steve Jobs from a distance. We were in the same room multiple times. He was usually surrounded by bodyguards and didn't stay in one place too long. His appearances were quick ins and outs to check that everything was up to his standards and, perhaps, to thank a few people along the way.

It was apparent to me and everyone else during those brief glimpses that the man was a genius with a larger-than-life aura. Unlike many other high-level business leaders, he had his hands in everything. Before a store opening, he inspected every minute detail. I remember watching him head up the flight of stairs surrounded by specially made Italian glass. He paused to stare at something. Everyone froze and became deathly silent as he deliberated. I don't remember what the problem was, but he caught something about the design that was a hair off. Nobody else had noticed it. Whatever it was, he insisted that they immediately redo the whole thing; he didn't care about the cost. He wasn't rude or disrespectful. He had a vision, was a total perfectionist, and had a gift for seeing things other people didn't.

We were going to rock the Apple store project, no matter what. We put everything we had into the assignment and caught lightning in a bottle: the thrilling moments of people absorbing the in-person Apple experience for the first time. This was a brand-new world for a generation of customers who were completely wowed by Steve Jobs' flagship storefront. There had never been anything like this in retail before. There were no shelves, no boxes, no big displays, no huge signage—just Apple products spread out on neat wooden tables for people to test drive. They could engage (or "play," as Jobs might have said) with the technology in an immaculately clean, beautifully lit environment that exuded elegance. Expertly trained staff in blue Apple Genius shirts and headsets catered to the needs of every guest.

Customers responded exactly as Jobs envisioned, giddily rushing through the store, flitting from one product to the next, and lining up at the registers. We may not have fully grasped it at the time, but this was historic. We took extra special care shooting and cutting the film to produce a gem that did complete justice to the groundbreaking event.

Our marketing contact at Apple couldn't have been more pleased with the result. She called me right away to say, "Listen, Steve Jobs really liked what you guys did with this video. He wants us to do a lot more work with you."

I thought, Holy crap, we did it! We pulled it off! We impressed him!

What more could we have asked for? We became a trusted Apple production vendor. We were a young company doing our thing and suddenly—during the worst economy in years—the floodgates were bursting open.

We had a mantra about this relationship: Don't fuck it up. This was a once-in-a-lifetime opportunity, and the slightest misstep could cause it to go away. We had to come through on their new projects, which included shooting Apple store openings all over North America, Europe, and Asia (where there were probably over two dozen alone). This meant hiring a whole team—scaling our business to handle one precious account. For a hundred or so days a year, we had crews spread across various continents working around the clock. We delivered stellar work over and over for years without any issues.

We must have done hundreds of content pieces for Apple over the years; no project was too big or too small. When they needed us, we jumped. We continued to cover store openings, product launches, and various other projects. We knew we were in an enviable position working with the most innovative company in the world.

We also recognized that this incredible ride wasn't going to last forever. As David Bowie said, "The end comes when the infinites arrive." I have no idea what that means, but I think it's a great way to end this chapter.

Chapter Five

Fifty Feet of Crap in the Moneyball Era

> I LOVE SPORTS. I LOVE ANIMALS. I LOVE KIDS. I WANT TO SAVE THE WORLD. SO HOW DO I COMBINE THOSE THINGS? I DON'T KNOW.
> —JOAN JETT

I'm a big baseball fan. Most baseball advertising work falls into the categories of existing footage and small pieces of live action or graphics. Not super exciting and usually derivative. It's the type of work WSF hadn't pursued in the past.

All that changed in February 2004 when my friend Kevin Gammon, Creative Director at McCann advertising in San Francisco, called me and asked, "Hey, Jonathan, do you think you might be interested in directing a campaign?"

Kevin had me hooked from just that one question. He had a reputation as a concept guy—a major talent who was breaking the mold. His team had already won a ton of awards using comedy in spots that integrated athletes to promote their organizations.

He filled me in on all the details and I flew out to Arizona, where he set my team up to shoot some commercials with several Oakland A's players during spring training. Why was I so eager and excited to participate in this production? In addition to trusting Kevin and wanting to work with him, I was aware that the A's team had risen during a pivotal time in baseball history: the famed Billy Beane era, which was made famous a few months earlier in Michael Lewis's bestselling book *Moneyball*. (The film adaptation, which starred Brad Pitt and Jonah Hill, was released several years later, in 2011.)

At the time, the A's suffered from the same dilemma as my team, the New York Mets: How do you create a winning Major League baseball team if you don't have a big bankroll to sign up big stars like the New York Yankees? In the later film, Billy Beane (Pitt) describes the problem in the rawest terms possible: "There are rich teams and then there are poor teams. Then there's fifty feet of crap. And then there's us."

The point: You need to find other ways to win. Billy Beane did something different and introduced a revolutionary concept. He hired an expert at computer algorithms to figure out what combination of talent would translate to wins. With Art Howe at the helm as manager, the team featured a group of hand-selected players who had a certain unique chemistry: Scott Hatteberg, Eric Chavez, Barry Zito, Tim Hudson, Mark Mulder, David Justice, Jeremy Giambi, and many others.

The day before the shoot, which happened to be the night of the Super Bowl, we met with a client—an executive with the A's—at the preproduction meeting. "Hey, Jonathan," he began.

"Barry Zito would love to have you and your team over to his house to watch the game with him. He wants to hang out and get to know you before the shoot."

I was like a five-year-old kid trying to act cool on the first day of kindergarten. At the time, all Major League players were larger-than-life to me, so I was starry-eyed. A chance to watch the Super Bowl at star pitcher Barry Zito's house? Hell, yeah! I ran out to the guys on my crew, grabbing them one by one to tell them about the rare invite. They were as giddy with excitement as I was. It felt surreal.

A few hours later, the exec returned to the meeting and lowered the boom. "Hey, Jonathan, I'm so sorry to do this to you . . . but I spoke to Barry, and unfortunately, he said it's not going to work out for the Super Bowl tonight. I'm so sorry. I hope you guys don't mind."

I was crushed. Somehow, I sucked it up. "Of course, no problem at all, these things happen. I totally understand."

I dreaded having to burst the bubble of all those guys who had their hearts set on hanging out with Barry Zito to watch the Super Bowl. With my head lowered, I pulled the guys aside and gave them the bad news. What a freaking disappointment. Now I felt like the five-year-old boy who traipsed to the candy store, only to find out they were out of his favorite candy.

I don't know who had chosen our shitty hotel, but man, it was depressing. It was in a corporate park in the middle of nowhere. My team and I figured we'd watch the game together on the TV in the hotel restaurant/bar. It seemed like a letdown, but we didn't have time to plan anything better.

Later that evening, we sat down at a table and ordered drinks. Suddenly, a member of our group pointed out PGA champion golfer Fuzzy Zoeller as he stepped into the bar/restaurant. By sheer coincidence, the PGA Tour was in town the same weekend. He sat down at the bar by himself.

The guys and I figured, "What the hell? What can we lose? He's all alone and probably wants some company."

We called out to him: "Hey, Fuzzy! Come over and watch the game with us!"

"Sure!" he exclaimed.

Two minutes later, he was at our table and already the life of the party. We drank and laughed before, during, and after the game. He couldn't have been funnier or more pleasant. It turned out that Fuzzy Zoeller was a fair trade for Barry Zito.

The next day, we went straight to business. We had just a few days to shoot eight commercials. We knew we had to work fast and get everything right. We didn't have a big budget and had to assume the baseball players were on tight schedules with plenty of other commitments.

Right from the start, I knew this A's team was something special and was honored to collaborate with them. I spent many hours working directly with Barry Zito, Scott Hatteberg, Eric Chavez, Mark Mulder, and Tim Hudson. They were a remarkable group of guys. They were in a great mood, as it was early in spring training and the players seemed to truly like each other and have fun hanging out together.

The goal was to create a whole bunch of funny, innovative spots to promote the Oakland A's team and brand. The advertiser wanted the fans to get quirky glimpses of the athletes that would generate excitement and fill the stadium seats.

The players couldn't have been more professional. Baseball stars and other athletes are at times in a rush to get in and out of commercial shoots and phone in their performances. This was far from the case with the A's. All the players were exceptional. They batted creative ideas around and always seemed to agree with each other and express encouragement.

Barry Zito was especially on the ball, as it were. We'd do take after take, and then he would insist on doing it over again: "No, no, no . . . I'm not done. I'm sure I could do better." He wasn't being challenging at all; he truly wanted to be sure the result turned out great.

In one of the spots, Hudson, Chavez, and Hatteberg were pranking one of their rookie teammates. They dressed him up in a goofy black suit with ping pong balls attached to it from top to bottom and told him he was going to be in a new video game. Of course, the video game was just a ruse to make the rookie look silly. The only problem was that we didn't have time to find an extra to play the role of the videographer. We asked around for a volunteer, but no one stepped forward, so I raised my hand and said, "Sure, I'll do it!"

"You're in!" Randy, the director, declared.

It took two hours to do the shoot, during which you can plainly see me standing behind a video camera. I was scared shitless. I'm a lot more comfortable behind the camera than I am in front of it. I prayed the entire time that I wouldn't fuck it up. Between takes, though, Hudson, Chavez, and Hatteberg were unbelievably cool with me. They shared hilarious problems and stories—the kind only professional baseball players could tell. I cracked little jokes whenever there was a lull. My head was in the clouds when they said, "Hey, you're a funny guy!"

In another classic spot—one in which I did not play a role—Zito and Hudson are warming up and throwing balls like they're in a gun-firing range. They launch balls one after another, harder and faster each time. As a viewer, we don't really know what's happening until the end. Hudson is presented with his pitching target sheet: All the balls have struck dead center. Pretty good, right? Then Zito is shown his target sheet: His balls are arranged to form the letter Z in the center (obviously, to represent his last name). Simple, smart, and hilarious.

I ended up meeting most of the A's team, including manager Art Howe and Billy Beane himself. Billy didn't look anything like Brad Pitt. He's taller, lankier, and has darker hair.

According to Kevin, though, Brad captured his mannerisms. Recently, Kevin said to me, "I vividly remember sitting down with Billy before we started. He took out a can of Copenhagen, snapped it open, took a big gulp, and swallowed. Then he put his feet up, and asked, 'You ever see Sports Center? Their commercials are awesome. I want my commercials to be as good as that.'"

A few weeks later, Billy personally told Kevin that he liked the commercials. They made him laugh. In our minds, he couldn't have offered a greater compliment.

Those spots captured a moment in time when the A's were the hottest thing in baseball. Other agencies have since tried to imitate it—such as some commercials with the Giants—but they couldn't hold a candle to what WSF did with McCann and that incredible team. At least that's my story and Kevin's—and we're sticking to it.

Chapter Six

Stepping Over Bodies at The Bowery

CBGB WAS A WILD PLACE . . . THE FIRST TIME I EVER PLAYED THERE WAS IN 1987, I THINK, WITH MY HARDCORE BAND, SCREAM. AND I REMEMBER THE CRAZIEST THING [ABOUT] THAT CLUB WAS THAT YOU COULD BE IN FRONT OF THE STAGE, AND IT COULD BE LOUDER THAN ANY SHOW YOU'VE EVER BEEN TO IN YOUR LIFE. BUT IF YOU WERE IN THE BACK OF THE CLUB AT THE BAR, YOU COULD SIT AND HAVE A CONVERSATION WITH SOMEONE. IT WAS THE WEIRDEST THING TO ME.
—DAVE GROHL

When I started at Washington Square Films, the office was in the heart of Greenwich Village, the home of Washington Square Park and the NYU campus. We were right next to where Joey Ramone lived on University Place and 10th Street. We had the lower level—literally below ground—of an old brownstone apartment building, which made it feel like an underground newspaper. Through the window, we were watching the world go by from the knees down. We even had our own little backyard. People lived in the apartments above us. It was a fun and cool place to work.

My division was on a roll. The Apple account was huge for us, and soon we had regular work with several major brands. One of the most fun accounts was working with Verizon on their memorable "Can you hear me now?" campaigns featuring Paul Marcarelli.

The entirety of WSF was firing on all cylinders; commercial production was just one piece. The management division was growing, while the films kept getting bigger and bigger. We added some incredible directors to our stable. The award nominations poured in: Academy Awards, Emmy Awards, Sundance, Cannes, etc. We had to add people to our staff, and our office space began to feel tight.

Josh began to scope out neighborhoods for a new office location. One thing I learned about Josh is that he has a sixth sense about things. He has an uncanny knack for anticipating the future and seeing things other people don't. He also knows what feels right for him and the business. The day came when he announced his plans to the staff. "It's really exciting—we're looking at the Bowery," he said. "It's the city's next up-and-coming neighborhood."

The reactions were not exactly what Josh had hoped for, ranging from skeptical to terrified. No one believed a word of what he was saying. In their eyes, the Bowery was a shithole to be avoided and several levels down from where we were comfortably situated. They didn't think the area was going to improve in a million years.

The Bowery roughly covers Chatham Square at Park Row, Worth Street, and Mott Street in the south; in the north, it reaches Cooper Square at 4th Street. Historically, the Bowery was never exactly known for anything stylish, romantic, or attractive from a business or real estate standpoint. It was a place marked by prostitution, gangsters, and slum living conditions. The neighborhood was the setting for the tragic Theodore Dreiser novel *Sister Carrie*. The closest Hollywood connection was the series of *Bowery Boys* plays and later film comedies from the late 1930s to late 1950s starring Huntz Hall and Leo Gorcey.

For the first decade of our current century, the Bowery continued to be sketchy and rough around the edges with a fair share of crime. So, it was understandable that my WSF colleagues were wary of our trading in this terrific place in the Village for some dumpy flea trap in a war zone.

Josh, however, knew in his gut that the Bowery was going to be the next hot spot in the city and its value was going to shoot through the roof. He bought 310 Bowery, situated off First Street.

While interior building renovations were taking place, Josh decided it was time for the WSF team to head off on a class field trip by foot to visit the new space. While his face was beaming in delight at the potential, nearly everyone else was horrified. Jaws dropped the moment we reached the neighborhood. The area was run-down and gross, infested with rats and roaches. Everywhere we looked were shady characters, pawnshops, and flophouses. On the sidewalk, we practically had to sidestep or hop over dead bodies.

I had a different reaction from my colleagues. No, I wasn't crazy about the rats, roaches, or dead bodies, either. But when I saw that CBGB was diagonally across from the building Josh had purchased as our new digs, I couldn't care less whose corpses were lying around. I nearly burst with excitement. This music venue was my home away from home, and I would have done anything to be situated there. I couldn't believe I was going to work so close to my sacred place.

The tour inside the building didn't receive a much better reception from the team. While my mind was still lost in a blissful CBGB fog and I saw potential for a much bigger office space, my coworkers were rolling their eyes at the hollowed-out walls and gaping holes in the floor.

The renovations were completed, we moved in, and everything turned out great. It was spacious and beautiful. Best of all, my office window overlooked CBGB—what a gift! I couldn't wait to arrive in the morning every day, put my bag down, and look at the sign across the street even before I turned my computer on. I would get goosebumps each time. It never grew old. I had incredible memories of all the amazing shows I attended there.

As it turned out, we settled into the area reasonably well. No WSF employees or clients were harmed while moving about in the Bowery or from tripping over those dead bodies.

I only recall one dangerous incident. A deranged guy covered with tattoos from head-to-toe entered our office and started threatening people. I don't know if he was an escapee from a mental institution, on drugs, homeless, or all three, but the danger was real; he was a Charles Manson–level nutjob. But the intruder picked the wrong day to show up and cause trouble. Our office manager at the time—who happened to be a double black belt in jujitsu—was present in the office. Let's just say he made the guy an offer he couldn't refuse, kicking his crazy tattooed butt out onto the street.

Meanwhile, Josh again proved he was a master prognosticator. The dead bodies were carted away, and one by one the neighborhood began to change. Condemned buildings came down like a row of accordions. Every day, it seemed, those eyesores were replaced by upscale condos. The ritzy Bowery Hotel drew in a major celebrity element. Designer Patricia Field opened her boutique store right next to our building. Other cool stores and Michelin-starred restaurants popped up. Soon enough, everything in the area had upgraded, except for one dilapidated flophouse, which charged $6 a night. An elderly lady tenant—who somehow had a long-term rental lease—was the sole holdout. It took a while, but eventually she caved into the pressure of a large buyout and that building was razed as well. The contractors couldn't wait to get that condo up in its place; it felt like it showed up the next day. Suddenly, we heard that this new building was the hottest property in New York and Hollywood star Anne Hathaway had just moved in.

When Whole Foods took up the corner space, the neighborhood's fate was sealed: Yuppie hell had officially broken loose! The Bowery suddenly became the "in" place to be.

It seemed as if every day I caught another celebrity sighting. I'd often see David Byrne riding around on his bicycle. I spotted Sarah Jessica Parker and Jonah Hill on a few occasions. The biggest star I saw of them all? David Freaking Bowie.

During an eclipse, the Bowery streets filled up with people in sunglasses looking up at the sky. I remember standing there in my shades hanging out with some people from my office when a guy tapped me from behind. "Hey, do you mind if I borrow your glasses? Just for a second."

I turned around to face actor/comedian Seth Rogen. My sunglasses immediately came off. "Sure, no problem!"

On paper, my commute to work was easy. The express trains from Fairfield to Grand Central Station were about an hour and twenty minutes. I'd hop on the Downtown 6 Train and get off at Bleecker Steet and Lafayette. My office was a three-minute walk from the subway stop.

On a good day, it would take under two hours for me to get from my house to my office. Then again, it seemed as if there were always problems on Metro-North: bad weather, electrical outages, delays, cancellations, broken trains, no heat, no air conditioning, obnoxious passengers, etc. The worst trains were the ones in the late hours after I had a long day of shoots or meetings or had been attending a dinner or some other event. After 11:30 p.m., anything goes. People drunk and puking. People having sex. People fighting. People throwing food and garbage. Good times. The conductors didn't give a shit.

In the days of the bar car—which are now long gone—it was a total shit-show. It stank to high heaven. People were drinking just to get totally fucked up. When they reached their stops, they'd fall off the train and hobble to their cars. I have no idea how many of them ended up in drunk driving accidents.

There was always one overly eager woman in the middle of the bar car, surrounded by a dozen wasted guys. She loved the attention, and the guys would be all over her. It was kind of pathetic.

The trains on Wednesday—matinee day in the city—drove me out of my fucking mind. You had all these loud-mouthed yentas talking at a such a loud decibel at 7:00 a.m. while the regular commuters like me were desperately trying to get some shuteye.

Coming home on matinee days—oh my God. The worst. I'd have to put up with enormous families with the parents lugging shopping bags, toys, and strollers while the kids were running around screaming at the top of their lungs, no rules whatsoever.

After a while, the long commute to and from the city every day in "the iron coffin" does take its toll on you. It can be exhausting. But I guess it was all worth it in the end. I loved the office, the Bowery neighborhood, and my window view to the CBGB marquee sign (which, unfortunately, is now gone). I also enjoyed the work itself, which was about to cross over into another huge passion area of mine . . .

Chapter Seven

The Gift of Schillervision

I'M A CULTURE VULTURE, AND I JUST WANT TO EXPERIENCE IT ALL.
—DEBBIE HARRY

Imagine the following scenario: A director hired to shoot a commercial for a major corporation shows up at preproduction to meet the client for the first time. The director is wearing dark shades and holding a cane. When the executives appear to greet the director, they are shocked to see the director place his hand on an assistant's shoulder and lead him to an opposite corner where no one is standing.

The execs are both stunned and horrified, not knowing what to say or do. Everything is heading straight down the crapper. Their minds are racing . . .

Oh my God, he's blind as a bat!

How can a blind director shoot a commercial?!

We just invested a shit ton of money in this guy and careers are on the line!

What can we say to him in this situation?

The director then roamed haphazardly around the office, banging into furniture and people while saying silly things along the way. This would continue for several minutes to see how long he could get away with the routine without breaking character. Yes, this was all just a hilarious comedy routine that had everyone—especially the relieved clients and me—cracking up.

Only one comic genius was daring and clever enough to concoct such crazy schemes like this: the great Tom Schiller. Of course, Tom did gags like these back in the mid to late 2000s when social norms were different. He recently said to me that he wouldn't attempt to do such politically incorrect things, such as act like a blind man, today.

Tom was one of the original writers on *Saturday Night Live* back in 1975, and he appeared as a cast member for one year. He became something of a legend for his funny and often touching short films on *SNL* in segments titled "Schiller's Reel" and "Hidden Camera" (commercials that became dubbed "Schiller Visions"). Tom had some big shoes to fill, as he took on the short film mantle from legends Albert Brooks and Gary Weis.

One of Tom's most famous shorts, "Don't Look Back in Anger" from 1978, involved an elderly John Belushi visiting the graves of his fellow SNL cast members in the distant future. (Ironically, Belushi was the first of them to pass away, just four years later.) In another, "La Dolce Gilda," Tom did a sendup of Italian filmmaker Federico Fellini's *La Dolce Vita* with Gilda Radner.

In the mid to late 2000s, WSF was on the hunt for a strong comedy director to shoot commercials. We started to shop around for someone and heard about a talented director, Tom Schiller, who had something of a reputation for, shall we say, unpredictable behavior. I loved his previous work, which included the "Real Men of Genius" Budweiser commercials. I also heard bits and pieces about his antics with clients and on sets and didn't quite know what to make of them.

I decided to meet with him in person and judge for myself. We shook hands and hit it off right away. He was the nicest guy in the world. He also happened to enjoy spontaneously goofing around. We signed him up and went on our first assignment about a month later.

I remember standing with him in an advertising agency's lobby when I received a phone call. "Listen, Tom, I'm really sorry—this call is really important. I have to take it. Stand right here. I'll just be a minute."

I stepped away for sixty seconds to handle the call when a security guard tapped me on the shoulder. "Hey, that guy who came in with you . . . can you tell him to stop running around our lobby as fast as he can? He's distracting the employees."

Sure enough, Tom was racing around the lobby like someone on speed. I knew it was all just a put-on for a harmless laugh. He spontaneously did stuff like that to entertain people or just keep them on their toes. It was all in good fun.

Tom usually started commercial shoots with some offbeat gag to lighten the mood. He told me, "Whenever we shot in Canada I played 'O Canada,' the Canadian National Anthem.

I also always did a safety speech for the cast and crew before the shoot began. I asked everyone to drop their heads to 'say the prayer' before starting the shoot. I recited some gibberish that sounded like a cross between mock-Hebrew and pig Latin. Some people took it seriously."

The "safety speech" requires a bit of an explanation. He would address the cast and crew about safety protocols by talking into a colorful plastic toy, a Radio Shack karaoke hand-held microphone. Sometimes he'd play ridiculous mood music in the background on a cheap cassette player as he spoke. He would end by saying that prizes were going to be handed out at the end of the shoot to those who best represented the safety protocols. (We'll get to that part a bit later . . .)

Most people got the joke and appreciated the humor, but there was one person in particular who didn't: actor William Shatner, who was offended by Schiller's routine before a Kellogg's shoot and described it as "juvenile." Schiller's response today is classic: "I was glad to have irked Kirk."

Now we get to the safety prizes, which Schiller awarded at the last minute at the end of each shoot. He would usually spread out the "winners" among the hardest-working people in the different departments: hair and makeup, craft service, the gaffers, the grips, and so on. (They were specifically not intended for people like me.) The honors were announced for inane things like "making the cables safe to not trip on." The prizes varied a bit, although there were usually some regular things in the mix of oddball items: iPods, talking toy parrots, and remote-control model helicopters. After a while, regulars on the set (including myself) looked forward to finding out who won the safety prizes and why. Tom made the process a blast.

As for the commercial shoots themselves, Tom was always the epitome of professionalism. Every final product ended up being incredibly entertaining. We did commercials for Meijer supermarket chain, the New York Lottery, McCormick spices, the Salvation Army/Red Cross, Discovery Channel/Shark Week, and more. I'll let Tom himself describe three memorable ones:

- **U.S. Mail:** *There was a U.S. mail spot we shot where a dog was supposed to lick an envelope shut. We achieved this by smearing butter on the envelope flap. The dog absolutely loved it and licked it heartily. A little too heartily. I never realized dogs loved butter so much!*
- **Lucky Supermarket:** *I loved this spot where we see the employees checking in on a timeclock at the beginning of the day when, suddenly, a whole apple tree appears and punches in with its branches.*
- **Optimum Online:** *We had the opportunity to re-create the set from* The Dating Game *TV show. I couldn't believe how realistic it turned out.*

While recalling these experiences, Tom said, "On a personal level, I'm so proud of the work we produced together."

I'm deeply flattered that he had some kind things to say about me as well: "Jonathan, you were always a pleasure . . . the consummate professional and could always be counted on to attend to every detail of the production, in addition to being a likable and skillful intermediary to the clients. I have nothing but good memories of collaborating with you during my tenure at Washington Square."

Chapter Eight

Sonic Youth and the Last Days of CBGB

MY MIND IS TURNING INTO KIND OF A FINE GELATINOUS BALL OF PEPPER.
—THURSTON MOORE

Have I mentioned how much I loved CBGB and seeing the awning through my office window every day? I have so many fond memories of shows I'd attended there back in the 1980s and '90s, including The Talking Heads, Patti Smith, Blondie, Sonic Youth, and Television. I must have seen the Ramones at least a half dozen times there, and their performances were the ones that stood out the most. They were a unique band with so much attitude: the same punk look with bangs over their eyes and long hair down the back and dressed in leather, tight jeans, T-shirts, and lace-up sneakers. The group would go through their two- to three-minute punchy songs without much dialogue among themselves or with the audience.

The irony is that, although CBGB was iconic and one of my favorite places in the world, in my opinion, it wasn't the best venue to see music. While it had a ton of character, the acoustics and views weren't great. The seating area blocked some standing room, and you had to arrive super early and sidle up close to feel the intimacy and fully enjoy the show and music. The CBGB Gallery, located right next door, was tiny and featured more obscure bands, but the floor was more open with much better sight lines to the stage.

CBGB's shortcomings as a venue take nothing away from its iconic status. This is probably going to sound strange, but it was worth going to a show there even if you didn't like the band playing that night, just to experience the bathroom with all the wild graffiti on top of graffiti. Not to mention the scantily clad punk girls with nose rings in tight leather outfits that left nothing to the imagination.

Another big attraction was the element of danger. When I went to shows with my friends, our mindset was *get in, don't get mugged, and get the hell out*. And, yeah, we did get mugged a couple of times. In that sense, it was a shitty place back then, both inside and out. Everywhere you looked, people were doing drugs. Fistfights were a common occurrence. I didn't involve myself in any of those things, but man, it was a great scene for people watching. All this action predated my collecting phase and, of course, cell phones. I wish I'd had the prescience of mind to have brought a guitar (or something else) for band members to sign or a camera to take cool shots of all the crazy stuff that went down.

I'm detailing all this stuff in this chapter to build up to how CBGB was already starting to face a steady decline shortly after WSF moved across the street. They just weren't getting the same level of talent anymore.

In June 2006, however, something monumental happened that blended my passion for music with the job I love. Braden King, one of our directors, was hired to direct a live show for Sonic Youth—who happened to be among my favorite bands—at CBGB. Jem Cohen (a legendary documentarian) and Sam Levy (who later became well-known for his work on *Lady Bird*) were recruited as cinematographers. Legendary punk photographer David Godlis was brought in to capture the moment in pictures.

Sonic Youth had made history playing there in June 1988 and again on July 3, 1992, in what became known as a "secret show," so this was something of a return to glory for them. The event wasn't open to the public, but a sizable crowd was in attendance—including me, of course. The band performed two amazing songs that ended up being cut into music videos: "Do You Believe in Rapture?" and "Reena." Seeing the band up close and experiencing the whole event as it unfolded was unbelievable. For me, it was the equivalent being on the rooftop with the Beatles as they performed songs for the *Let It Be* film. The video "Do You Believe in Rapture?" was released in August 2006.

Braden King recently described it this way to me: "I wanted Jem's footage to have a sort of nostalgic feel to it and a tinge of timelessness . . . We created it as kind of like a dream or a memory of all the great shows we'd all ever been to. It was like how I wanted it to feel—and how you remember a concert later. The concept was like, 'We'll shoot the whole show and then we'll pull clips and put them to the music in ways that aren't exactly in sync—but they are more expressive.'"

A couple of months later, on October 15, 2006, Patti Smith performed at the final show at CBGB before it officially closed. I wasn't clued in to it happening at the time. I may have been traveling for work or just wasn't dialed in the way I should have been. I wish I had been. Why hadn't I taken pictures of the inside while I had a chance—or at least one photo of the building's awning, which I saw through my window every weekday? I guess I took it for granted that CBGB would always be there. Until it wasn't.

Today, what had been CBGB is now John Varvatos men's clothing store. CBGB Gallery has been turned into a Patagonia chain store. Talk about a comedown from what I used to see through my window!

That's not to say the neighborhood has completely buried its punk roots. A street at Bowery and Second Street in the East Village pays tribute to the Ramones with the sign "Joey Ramone Place." The corner of Bleecker Street and Bowery features a beautiful rotating mural of the greatest bands who made history in the area: the Ramones, Bad Brains, Blondie, and many others. I love walking past it, as it brings back all kinds of great memories.

A few years later, I traveled to Cleveland with a production crew for a commercial shoot and went to check out the Rock and Roll Hall of Fame. There, on display, was the physical CBGB awning I'd seen through my window every day. I thought, You've got to be kidding me!

Still, I'm grateful that it hadn't been destroyed or purchased by some crazed fan who would hang it in their basement. Of course, the latter is exactly what I would have done if I'd been given the chance.

Chapter Nine

The Green Monster Invades Third Avenue

EVERYONE THINKS I'M A WIMP AND EVEN MY OWN BAND HATES ME. OH, WELL. I GUESS I'LL JUST FLIP 'EM THE BIRD!
—FRANK BLACK (AKA BLACK FRANCIS)

Imagine you're a New Yorker wearing your Yankees cap and you're happily strolling along the city streets on a beautiful spring day when . . . suddenly . . . you pass by a gigantic replica of the Green Monster.

"The Green Monster?! In my city?! WTF?!"

Yes, you read that correctly: A humongous facsimile of the famed green outfield wall from Fenway Park in Boston was once erected on a Manhattan block. I'm proud to say I played a minor role in creating this incredible stunt.

Let's backtrack to the beginning, May 1, 2015. Major League baseball season had started just a few days earlier. Benjamin Moore and their agency had come up with the brilliant idea of marketing paint in the color of every Major League baseball stadium. Red Sox fans, for example, could purchase green paint that was an exact match to the Green Monster, recreating the feel of America's oldest ballpark in their own basements (or wherever).

The Martin Agency reached out to me about WSF producing a video to promote this new line of paint colors. The concept: Build the Green Monster in the place where it's despised the most and see how New Yorkers react. It was fun, innovative, controversial, and easy to grasp. Making this happen wasn't going to be so simple. At first, I thought the producer was kidding—but they were serious about it. We accepted the challenge and moved forward. While I thought the idea was hilarious—especially since I happen to be a legendary Yankees hater—I worried about how the hell we were going to pull this off.

First things first. We had to find the perfect site, which we did: an empty lot on the corner of Third Avenue and 21st Street. Next, we needed to order enough building materials to construct an authentic Green Monster wall on the street and assign a crew to put it together—super fast.

A million ideas raced through my mind as we assembled all the pieces. The agency came up with the idea of hiring the right "voice" of the Green Monster to stand hidden behind the wall and taunt people on the other side. It had to be someone with a spot-on thick Bostonian accent. We landed just the right guy: comedian and actor Lenny Clarke, who was perhaps best known for his role on the TV show *Rescue Me*.

We sorted out all the details of the shoot, but I realized that we had to do everything all in one day. I knew that, if we were to construct the Green Monster at night in New York City, it would never survive until daybreak the next morning. There was no doubt in anyone's mind that word would get around among Yankees fans and they would show up in droves to smash it down long before we could shoot the commercial.

At the crack of dawn on May 1, 2015, the trucks rambled in and dumped a ton of building material on the sidewalk. A large crew went to work rapidly assembling the wall, finishing the project in just three or four hours.

I couldn't believe it: The Green Monster was right there in Manhattan. You could easily be fooled into thinking it was the real deal, transplanted from Fenway. The paint color was the perfect shade of green. The scoreboard displayed the Red Sox beating the Yankees 4-2 in the third inning of a game—with the hashtag #MONSTEREVERYWHERE emblazoned next to it. When I looked at it, I could picture Manny Ramirez or Carl Yastrzemski catching a ball smacked against it or Carlton Fisk slamming his historic home run a mile over it in the 1975 World Series.

Yankees fans who happened to be in the area were totally caught off guard. The hostility began right away. They started kicking and yelling at the wall and shaking it long before the cameras were rolling.

Now came the real work: setting up the commercial and getting the shoot done before there was a real riot and the wall would get knocked down. Lenny Clarke didn't have a script—and he didn't need one. We couldn't have found a better improvisor voice for the Green Monster. He could think on his feet and ad-libbed the whole thing for several hours. The gag was that he could see the people on the other side of the wall and approaching it, but they were unable to see him. He dove in headfirst, as it were, singing the fan chant with organ music: "Let's go Red Sox, Let's go Red Sox, Let's go Red Sox!"

Then the taunting began. Lenny shouted out to a guy passing by, "Hey, turn around, look at me! I'm the Green Monsta!"

"What are you doing here in New York?" the puzzled pedestrian asked.

"Driving people crazy!" Lenny replied.

A woman placed her nose up against the wall and sneered, "You're in the wrong city, buddy!"

"Hashtag: I don't care!" he fired back in a Boston accent.

A bearded guy with glasses in a green shirt was really pissed and shouted out all kinds of expletives we had to bleep over: "Boston, you can go fuck yourself!"

Another Yankees fan became threatening and wagged his finger at the wall: "I don't know how they put you here, in this city!"

A woman threatened to spit on it. And then she did.

Another young woman stood by the wall with her arms folded as she deliberated on how she was going deal with this insulting monstrosity attacking her beloved city.

"Maybe you should paint your bedroom in Green Monster, would you like that?" Lenny suggested. "I could come over!"

When someone went by while walking a couple of dogs, he quipped, "Don't let those dogs pee on me—get outta here!"

Lots of birds were flipped.

As a young Yankees fan stood in front of the wall trying to figure out what was going on, Lenny teased, "What do you think when I say the year 2004?"

He asked this question several times with other Yankees fans, except he added choking sounds afterward.

"Get outta here!" a Yankees fan recoiled. Another gave two "thumbs down."

We later piped in the Red Sox classic stadium theme song "Dirty Water" by the Standells. Lenny got really into it: "That's what I'm talking about!"

It didn't take long for a few Red Sox fans to show up and support the wall, singing and dancing along with the music. "Now you got it, now you're doing it—that's what the wall likes!" Lenny exclaimed.

CUT TO: A can of Benjamin Moore Green Monster paint being opened along with the music. Lenny continued to play his role with gusto, reciting a few familiar New Yorker words: "Listen, if you can make here, you can make it anywhere!"

The commercial draws to a close with a Yankees fan punching the wall and another warning for it to "Go back to Boston!"

Lenny had the last word: "All right. 2004!"

The spontaneous shoot worked perfectly. It was a long but wildly successful day. Some news crews reported on it and lots of videos went viral on social media. The people at Martin Agency and Benjamin Moore were thrilled with the result. It ended up winning a ton of awards, too, including the prestigious Cannes Lion.

If you loathe the Yankees as I do, check out the Benjamin Moore video on Facebook dated May 1, 2015. Or explore the hashtag #MonsterEverwhere.

If you happen to be a Yankees fan, I hope there are no hard feelings.

Oh, one last thing: The Yankees really do suck.

Chapter Ten

Henry, Beckham, and a Bag of Lay's

**THERE'S A BIT OF MAGIC IN EVERYTHING,
AND THEN SOME LOSS TO EVEN THINGS OUT.
—LOU REED**

It's hard for me to believe: Thirty years later and my career with the same company is going strong and we are producing some of our best work ever. Who knew that, when I first met Josh for coffee all those years ago, it would have led to so many great campaigns and such a longstanding, thriving business. I'm proud we continue to be as creative and relevant as ever.

Another of my favorite highlights has been the opportunity to work with legendary ad man Gerry Graf, whom I've known since the early 2000s. Back in the day, we created a hilarious commercial for Raid floral scent in which a cockroach with a Woody Allen-esque nerdy voice is in the throes of death ("I see the light . . .") while running in a field of daffodils (when he is being zapped to death by Raid bug spray).

After Gerry co-founded his own company, SlapGlobal, in 2021, he called me to see if WSF would be interested in doing experiential-type work with PepsiCo's Frito-Lay division for a Lay's potato chip campaign. The concept—to shoot in Europe with French football (soccer for us Americans) great Thierry Henry unexpectedly popping up at people's homes. This sounded simultaneously daunting and exciting. We jumped on the opportunity right away, especially because one of our directors, Andrew Lane, specialized in handling such crazy hidden camera stunts.

In the commercial, Henry showed up unannounced at the front doors of fans' homes and asked if they had a bag of Lay's potato chips; if they did, he'd watch a game on their couch with them. The people frantically scavenged their homes to the tune of the Go-Go's song "We Got the Beat" while Henry waited at the door. One person came up empty. Another brought out potatoes, which caused Henry to crack up with laughter. Unfortunately, the lack of Lay's chips disqualified these fans, and Henry ran off to find another contender. Finally, a trio of teenagers presented a bag of Lay's to Henry, and he welcomed himself inside their living room. For the remainder of the commercial, Henry sat in the middle of the couch between the young fans and enjoyed the game while chomping on chips. A few quick cuts at the end showed the utter disappointment of the fans who missed out because they failed to produce a bag of Lay's to the star.

Boom! The commercial went viral. It won some Cannes Lion awards that year for best advertising. Everyone at SlapGlobal and PepsiCo was thrilled.

We didn't stop there. The goal, as it were, was to go even bigger for a follow-up "Chip Cam" campaign. Director Andrew Lane worked his magic yet again to pull off a live commercial in San Siro stadium in Milan, Italy, at a game in front of more than 70,000 fans. We took the star power to the next level by adding the one and only David Beckham alongside Henry. The pair announced to the packed stadium that they could have a rare opportunity to sit on a bench and watch the game side by side with these icons—if they had a bag of Lay's potato chips. The crew had under five minutes just prior to kickoff to find fans in the stands who had the right chips. The crowd went nuts, lighting up flares and smoke grenades and waving flags. The noise level was deafening. In the nick of time, the perfect father and teenage daughter team were identified with a bag of Lay's and ushered down to the field for a major seat upgrade. True to the promise, they were gifted the dream of watching the entire game on a bench sandwiched between two of their heroes. It was unbelievably cool to see the four of them interact like four old friends who shared a passion for the sport—and Lay's potato chips, of course.

This second commercial garnered even more acclaim and Cannes Lion awards than the previous one. The spots have been so successful that we have more celeb athlete surprises in the works. Collaborating with the people from SlapGlobal and PepsiCo is a dream.

All this achievement had been happening at the same time WSF produced *The Room Next Door*, by internationally acclaimed Spanish filmmaker Pedro Almodóvar and starring

Tilda Swinton, Julianne Moore, and John Turturro. The drama won the Golden Lion for best film at the 81st Venice International Film Festival in September 2024.

One sidenote about Gerry Graf. We've formed a bond outside our business relationship because we've both had to face family health crises. In his case, his oldest daughter, Sophie, had to endure leukemia during the height of the COVID-19 pandemic. Her younger brother, Gus, ended up being her bone marrow donor, which helped save her life. He also held a fundraiser at school, selling bracelets that said fuck cancer. (It's not an uncommon sentiment.) I'm happy to say that, as of this writing, Sophie has been cancer-free for nearly three years.

This leads us full circle back to the crux of my story when a simple dental issue turned my life upside down . . .

Chapter Eleven

Hey Doc, I Have a Bump On My Ass

> CANCER SOFTENED ME UP. I LIKE THE OLD ME BETTER. I LIKED BEING ANGRY. IT MADE ME FEEL STRONG.
> —JOHNNY RAMONE

Remember when I boasted that I'd beat cancer? Let's go back to the specific words I used: *You can go fuck yourself*...

Well, life can be a bitch—and there is no bigger bitch in the world than cancer. Just when I thought I was out of the woods, my own words ended up biting me in the ass. Literally.

I went through hell during the second half of 2021. My mother had passed away, the COVID-19 pandemic was ongoing, and a seemingly innocuous discomfort in my sinuses turned out to be lymphoma: stage 4 cancer. After struggling at first to receive the proper medical care, I cut through the red tape and made it into Memorial Sloan Kettering Cancer Center (MSK). I had one of the best cancer specialists in the world, who put me through the wringer with chemo treatments: R-CHOP and then R-ICE. Six months and roughly seven cancer treatments later, I was told I was cancer-free.

To say I was itching to get back out into the world would be a major understatement. I was aching to be free and travel again with my family. I was jumping out of my skin to attend concerts and once again eat at great restaurants. I was desperate to resume working full throttle at WSF and do what I do best with my clients in person and on production sets.

Believing I had cancer beat, my family and I planned a vacation over the holidays in December 2022 to Palm Springs in Southern California. Then a month or so before the trip, I noticed something funky: a bump on my butt. I could no longer casually attribute health issues to my being a hypochondriac. Once you've gone through cancer, the antennae are always on the alert for something potentially wrong. My first thought was that it was a hemorrhoid or cyst—but what did I know? I'd never had anything like this, certainly not in this area. Just to be sure, I rushed to have it checked out.

I still had a VIP plan with my doctor, so I didn't have any difficulty setting up an appointment right away in New York City. My doctor examined it and said it was a cyst. Nothing to worry about. He added that, if it really bothers me, I could go to a colorectal doctor to have it checked out and possibly removed for peace of mind (or, um, bottom). This specialist arrived at the same conclusion: a cyst. He said it was no big deal to remove it, but since it wasn't any kind of real threat, it could wait until after my vacation.

So I went to Palm Springs for a pleasurable two weeks with my family—butt pain notwithstanding. We had the greatest time: lots of sun, amazing food, and an opportunity to explore new places like Joshua Tree National Park. The kids were in college and now had a much greater appreciation for the little things in life. We could finally exhale and enjoy something of a restart. I can only imagine the relief Mara felt coming through the other side of enduring my massive cancer treatments and all the traumas and side effects that went with them.

When we returned to Connecticut, reality set in right away with the New Year. The bump on my butt was swelling up and becoming even more painful. Then I started to notice bumps in the front area, too—right in my nut sack. There is nothing more chilling for a guy than having lumps and bumps on both sides down there.

First thing was first: I had to schedule the procedure with my colorectal doctor in New York City to get rid of the lump on my butt. Everything seemed fine afterward, and I dozed off. My eyes were half-open when I noticed the colorectal doctor standing over me. I didn't think anything of it and was barely even paying attention.

"Jon," the doctor began. "I've been doing this a long time. I must admit, I've never seen a tumor in this place before . . .."

Now I was fully awake. "What?"

"The lump we removed is definitely a tumor—not a cyst," he informed. "Based on your medical history, we need to run a battery of tests on it to determine if it's benign or not."

Shit. A tumor. This can't be good.

The recovery from this procedure wasn't exactly a walk in the park. My butt pain was excruciating all the time, especially when I had to sit down or do a number two. This meant that pretty much anything I did aggravated the area. Finding a comfortable sleeping position became a major challenge.

Meanwhile, as I was recovering from the procedure and panicking about the analysis of the butt tumor, I had to deal with the lumps in my nut sack—which were also worsening. Four or five days later, while Mara and I were in the car on our way to the urologist to have an ultrasound on my scrotum, I received a call from the colorectal doctor. The lab results were in.

I heard only one word: *lymphoma*.

Fuck—so much for being out of the woods.

I couldn't believe that so many competent, knowledgeable New York City doctors had been so wrong about that lump. We'd kicked the can down the road and now had to deal with the inevitable, having waited over a month and given the fuckwad lymphoma more time to grow and spread. Here's a no shit reality check that smacked me hard: Cancer is a formidable foe and can baffle the best of medical professionals, hiding and appearing however, wherever, and whenever it feels like.

Next, I had to deal with the test results on the scrotum lumps. You've probably connected the dots already and arrived at the obvious conclusion: They were lymphoma, too.

I had to dive right back into multiple rounds of chemo treatments—even more aggressive than before—this time to cover my entire pelvic region, where the cancer had become deeply embedded. Some of the sessions were in-patient, others out-patient. Both were brutal. There were tons of side effects. Nausea and hair loss were just the beginning. Taking a bite out of anything became painful in my jaw and face. Going to the bathroom was utter torment, like having the worst hemorrhoids on earth. I developed a complete intolerance to cold—in the middle of East Coast winter, no less. Any slight dip in temperature hurt like daggers. I wore multiple layers of clothing, as well as scarves and hats to cover myself up, but there was always something exposed—on my face or elsewhere on my body—that suffered from the chill.

The barrage of chemo was essential to clear my system of cancer for the next nightmare, which would take place in April: a stem cell transplant using my own cells. If there was even the slightest speck of cancer in my body, the doctors would have been unable to move forward with the subsequent treatment.

Flash forward a few weeks, after the poisonous chemo had been funneled in and out of my body, killing good and bad cells throughout my system. A PET scan showed that there was still cancer, so I was unable to have the stem cell transplant. The doctors had to pivot and decided that chimeric antigen receptor (CAR-T) was the best treatment option. By May, I was deemed ready for part two: a CAR-T cell transplant, which involved removing my cells and genetically modifying them to attack bad ones when they would be reintroduced into my body. I had to remain in-patient for about ten days. This was cutting-edge sci-fi medical shit and relatively new, but the doctors were optimistic about its effectiveness.

As I learned from the beginning, every good cancer treatment comes with a risk of nasty side effects. Welcome, cytokine release syndrome (CRS)! When this occurred, the genetically modified cells went rogue, releasing too many cytokines that hijacked my neurological system and sent me to the intensive care unit for five days that have mostly been lost to me forever. I barely remember a fucking thing that happened during this time; it was like my brain was extracted and transported somewhere else.

The way Mara describes it now, I was a human vegetable. While I could say words, I had no memory of anything—including her!—and couldn't pass a simple intelligence test that would be aced by a toddler. They asked me basic questions, such as count from one to ten backward or repeat simple sentences like "Today is a lovely day." They put a clock in front of me and told me to position the hands at a certain time. For the life of me, I was unable to do it. I couldn't name where I was or who was president. When I was asked, "Do you know what month it is?" I answered, "Massachusetts." Pure genius!

While I do not recall those specifics, I do remember my frustration. I touched my head and felt a skull cap device on me, tracking my brain waves. I was aware that I was a moron and screwing up. I also have a memory of Mara looking at me with what I interpreted as pity. It felt as if her emotions were all over her face: I can't believe what's happened to my husband.

I said something to her along the lines of "Stop looking at me like that. I know I can't answer these basic questions. I can't stand that you're looking at me with pity."

Miraculously, whatever intelligence I had gradually returned, which was a major relief to everyone—especially Mara and me. I knew where I was, recognized people, and counted backward from ten without any issue. I was barking out complaints like, "Get this damn thing off my head!" and "Yank this fucking catheter out of me!" which were good signs that I was returning to my usual cantankerous self. I recovered well enough to be moved out of the ICU.

By June, I was out of the woods with the side effects and detectable signs of cancer. Nobody was declaring victory, however. I had to continue with constant medical visits and do full scans every six months. It goes without saying that, throughout all this time, I was missing out on what was happening in terms of life's moments, both big and small. I was unable to go on the drives to and from college to help my kids with move-ins. Mara did a ton to support them, but both Alissa and Matt had to step up big time and handle things independently, which they did phenomenally well. I didn't spend nearly as much time with them as I would have liked, and I hardly ever saw my dogs, Smoke and Lacey.

My job was a godsend. Josh continued to be incredibly understanding and flexible about how, where, and when I worked. Although I was working remotely in a different capacity, I felt like I was still in the game. I was able to contribute and keep the wheels turning, thanks to Zoom meetings and my phone. Focusing on work helped keep me busy and retain my sanity. So did binge-watching TV shows with Mara, such as *Jury Duty* and *Banshee* (which is off-the-charts entertainment in terms of violence and sex, if you're into this sort of thing).

As the cliché goes, I was just taking things one day at a time. I consider myself to have been so lucky to have been surrounded by such incredible people: Mara, my sister Stefanie—whom, as I've mentioned, is an excellent caregiver type of person—and so many good friends from childhood, college, Fairfield, and work. People were frequently checking in to see how I was doing. This became even more important as I had to deal with yet another hundred-mile-an-hour curveball coming straight toward my head . . .

Chapter Twelve

I Think I Have a Headache

> THIS WHOLE THING HAS BECOME A PANTOMIME.
> —SID VICIOUS

I wasn't feeling too badly in February 2024 when I went in for a regularly scheduled PET scan. At the time, I was thinking that everything was going to turn out okay . . .

Ahem. I should have known better. For me, nothing was okay or stable. Every day, it seemed, I had to prepare myself for the next fucking nightmare.

The PET scan revealed cancer in the pelvis. Up until that time, I hadn't noticed anything off-base in that area, so this ended up being yet another shock. I entered an immunotherapy trial, which, as I recall, meant taking a simple pill. Within a week or two, my pelvic area was flooded with pain. I could barely walk. By April, the doctors realized this treatment wasn't working, and they switched to radiation. I ended up having something like eighteen rounds of radiation in the pubic area.

My condition initially caused serious doubts about my ability to attend our daughter Alissa's graduation from Ithaca in May. Somehow, I recovered enough to make it there, although I was far from perfect. Mara handled the long drive up there with some help from our son, Matthew. It wasn't comfortable, but there was no way I was going to miss the joy of our daughter's big day.

Some accommodations had to be made for me. College graduations can drag on, and I couldn't sit or stand for very long, so Mara arrived early and reserved seats. Once I was settled, everything went fine. I was so happy just to be there and incredibly proud of Alissa, who graduated Magna Cum Laude. We celebrated with two amazing dinners in the Ithaca area.

Next, it was back to my cancer reality. The good news was that the radiation blew out the cancer in the pelvis. The bad news was that a spot in my abdominal area had appeared, raising new concerns. I prequalified for a trial of CAR-T cell immunotherapy at the Dana-Farber Cancer Institute in Boston that was designed specifically for people who had already undergone this treatment.

On arrival at Dana-Farber toward the end of June, I went through the usual pretrial battery of tests to double-confirm that I qualified. Everything seemed to be going fine, and I was raring to go . . . until I casually commented to one of the doctors "I think I have a headache" while on my way out the door from one of the tests. Headaches were unusual for me; I rarely suffered from them. I described the headache as a "dull pain that would come and go," maybe a five or six on a scale of one to ten. I also admitted that I was having some difficulty expressing words.

By this point in my medical journey, no major or minor symptom was ever going to go untested, so on July 3, they pressed the pause button on initiating the treatment and ushered me in for a brain MRI. We were on our drive home for the July 4 holiday when I received a call from one of the doctors informing me that I no longer qualified for the treatment.

"Why not?" I asked.

I don't know how to tell you this, but the MRI results came in," he said, pausing. "The scan is positive for brain lymphoma."

This was another of those life-stopping moments for me, like years earlier when I was standing in the hallway of my house and was first informed that I had cancer. Cancer was totally fucking *me*, not the other way around.

Ironically, we later discovered that the second CAR-T cell treatment that I'd failed to qualify for was proven ineffective and subsequently shitcanned. It wouldn't have done anything to help me anyway!

After July, I went back to MSK for further testing. They did lumbar punctures, which is the same as a spinal tap—and just as horrible. Once the fluid has been extracted, they test it for cancer. I'd already had a few of these procedures, and you never get accustomed to them. Afterward, I experienced terrible headaches and vomited in my buddy's car on the way into New York for treatment. It was at this moment that Mara and I realized we needed a place to stay in New York City. The back-and-forth to Connecticut was too hard for both of us. The seed was planted for us to consider looking for an apartment in the city and living there full-time.

Yet again, I had to go back on chemo medication: a high dose of methotrexate IV. This drug has many applications, including the treatment of cancer and rheumatoid arthritis. The way it was phrased to me is that methotrexate is one of only a few drugs that break the blood brain barrier and make it north of the neck. If that sounds terrifying, it's because it is. I had to go into the hospital every two weeks because the drug messes with all your numbers. It's highly toxic, which means it must reach the brain with lightning speed and then clear right out of your body (via another drug). As with everything else, methotrexate comes with its own unique array of side effects. My blood numbers were impacted, and I experienced a lot of kidney and endocrine issues. Fun stuff.

Meanwhile, unrelated to the methotrexate, other issues cropped up. I had adrenal insufficiency—a condition in which the adrenal glands don't produce enough of the hormones cortisol and aldosterone—and had to go on IV hydrocortisone. Then I had major thyroid issues. As if that's not enough, I came down with diabetes insipidus, which isn't like regular diabetes, but made me feel crazy thirsty. I would stay up all night munching on ice and drinking water, which, of course, made me constantly pee.

After around the second dose of methotrexate, the doctors considered inserting something in my brain called an Ommaya reservoir. It's kind of like the port that goes into the chest, except that it gets placed in the brain to extract fluid. The thought was that this device would replace the need for my having frequent lumbar punctures while also doubling as a direct place in which to deposit the methotrexate.

Things did not go as planned. (When it's come to my health, when has anything ever gone according to the plan?) The New York electrical power grid happened to go down that day, wreaking havoc on the hospital. All the hospital alarms—including the ones in the patients' rooms—sounded off at the same time, so they had to shut them off. The Ommaya reservoir idea was postponed.

At the time, I wasn't supposed to get out of bed on my own, due to a high risk of falling. I don't recall having done this, but, in the middle of the night, I must have traipsed out of bed to go to the bathroom. As I mentioned, the hospital alarms had been turned off, so no one was aware of what I was doing. At some point, I wiped out and smashed my head. I was lying on the bathroom floor for a while—I have no idea how long—before someone noticed me.

The aftermath wasn't pretty. I had brain bleeding from the fall and was incoherent. Mara told me that when she arrived at the hospital the following morning, I barely recognized her.

As a precaution, the doctors put me on Keppra, an anti-seizure medication, although they didn't know if a seizure had caused the wipeout or not. The medication made me all kinds of loopy and delusional. Mara says I was like a dementia patient. I would repeat the same story ad nauseum. I babbled all kinds of grand ideas, including making a rap video and posting it on

TikTok. I even sent my sister on a mission to get candy props, like Nerds Gummy clusters. Man, imagine if I'd gone through with it—I bet it would have gone viral. In the annals of shitty ideas, this was right up there.

It was around this time that I started to become uncharacteristically emotional. I was crying all the time. Random doctors, nurses, psychiatrists, rabbis, priests, social workers—or whomever—would show up in my hospital room doing their rounds, and I'd just start weeping like a baby for no reason. I found out that this is yet another side effect of the medications and, once it starts, it's something that never completely goes away. It's the gift that keeps on giving.

My brain was so jumbled that I sent random unintelligible texts to Mara throughout the night. I suppose this wasn't helped by the fact that I was having trouble seeing; everything appeared to be dark. I can only imagine what she thought being on the receiving end of all that gibberish.

The one positive thing resulting from this ordeal is that I became obsessive about needing to get my story down on paper. I'd hit a total brick wall. I was going through the worst part of my life and couldn't even function. I didn't know if there was going to be a tomorrow for me.

A voice inside my fucked-up brain just kept repeating: I have to get this story out. The idea for this book, *F*ck Cancer*, started to take shape . . .

***

By early August, the head injury healed, and the focus returned solely on dealing with my brain tumor. The methotrexate IV continued every couple of weeks. Then came the most hopeful news I'd received in a long time: A new MRI revealed that the tumor was shrinking. The doctors did an about-face, deciding they didn't need to insert the Ommaya reservoir in my brain after all.

I ended up doing five cycles of methotrexate in total. They normally do eight, but as far as the doctors could see at the time, the disease was gone, so they were ready to blast me with chemo to clean me out in preparation for the next phase—an Allogenic stem cell transplant—on October 11.

Now I am not a religious guy, but this happened to fall on the Jewish High Holy Day of Yom Kippur. I saw this as a sign. Someone was looking down on me. The donor donated his cells on October 10, so we had to rock and roll the next day in the MSK building.

It turns out the donor was giving his stem cells in another building. Once they had collected enough cells from him, someone did their best O.J. Simpson to run over and get the volunteer's cells into my body ASAP. Afterward, I hung out for a few hours in the hospital and was then dismissed to go home.

The misery started about four days later. I was warned that my body might have a negative reaction adapting to the new stem cells. They weren't kidding. I passed out while doing my business in the bathroom and was admitted to the hospital, just to make sure everything was okay. They discharged me from the hospital, but the adverse effects continued. I won't get into all the gory details; let's just say I had some inclement bathroom activity.

I was a handful for Mara. I can't imagine how difficult it was for her to take care of me. I was physically drained and required constant care and monitoring. Even walking a few blocks to the hospital was becoming unmanageable. On one occasion, I started out okay but then couldn't go any further. Luckily, the Hospital for Special Surgery Main Hospital (known as HSS) was on the way and called MSK to send a wheelchair for me. We realized that this back-and-forth and home care was getting too hard for both of us and I had to be checked into the hospital.

Suddenly, my left arm started to hurt. Sure, why not my arm? Everything else in my body had been fucked up at one time or another, so why leave this limb out of the medical party?

At first, the arm looked perfectly normal. That night, however, it turned reddish/purple. The nurse drew dots on it with a blue Sharpie to measure for changes in size. Within a couple of days, it ballooned out over the blue boundaries, riding up my shoulder. The reddish/purple color kept worsening, too.

One of the doctors explained to me that it was some type of unidentifiable infection. If it were to get any worse, there was great risk of it spreading to my organs and becoming life-threatening. The talk led to the possibility of amputating my arm. This surgery would be high risk for me, since my platelets were basically at zero, which meant that I didn't have any ability to clot—an essential part of any healing process.

Talk about a shit-show. Which scenario was worse—dying from cancer, the swelling, or the after-effects of an amputated arm? As if I hadn't been in a dark enough place already with all the crap that was going on.

They pumped a ton of antibiotics into me, which didn't seem to be working quickly enough. A surgeon who checked on me said that, if it didn't improve by the next day, the arm was coming off. This shit was as real as it could get. I was terrified.

The next day, the arm showed miraculous improvement. The antibiotics were finally kicking in. Although there was some scarring and continued weakness in my arm, at least it would remain attached to my body. That was some freaking close call.

Not long after, engraftment—when transplanted stem cells establish themselves in the recipient's bone marrow and begin to produce new blood cells—also started to occur, which meant the transplant was cooperating and I could finally heal. Maybe . . .

***

We've reached February 2025 in my story, which means we're nearly caught up to present-day. I wish I could say everything was, to reference the David Bowie album, hunky dory. Far from it. Every day, it seems, I'm facing another shitstorm and have no idea what the future has in store.

Normally, the doctors do PET scans on me every 100 days or so to detect any sign of cancer. Before we reached that mark, I started to have headache flareups again. After a bout of vomiting, I went to Urgent Care, where they did an MRI. I was informed that the tumor was growing again in the same general area as when it first appeared. They decided to do the same treatment as last time—methotrexate—since it had already cleared the tumor once before.

After enduring two methotrexate cycles, I was feeling lightheaded and could barely get to appointments without being in a wheelchair. Pinpointing the cause was complicated by the fact that Mara and I had contracted the flu and my symptoms could have been related to that. At the same time, I was also experiencing numbness and tingling in my face. The doctors prescribed medication for this, but were suspicious about the headaches and weren't going to take any chances based on my history. Yet again, I was scheduled for an MRI, but my condition with the flu was so fucked up that I cancelled the MRI to go to Urgent Care. The MRI had to wait until the following Thursday morning—when it showed that the tumor was growing and the current treatment wasn't working.

The doctors decided it was time for a complete treatment change. I switched to a new medication, Imbruvica (the brand name for Ibrutinib), which isn't a chemotherapy drug. It works by inhibiting the enzyme Bruton's tyrosine kinase (BTK), which is part of a crucial signaling pathway in certain types of cancer, such as mine. Like the previous drug, it's one of the few things that passes that blood brain barrier and makes it north of the neck. Unfortunately, it doesn't work on everyone. As of this writing, I have small reason to be hopeful, as I feel a bit more energy. Time will tell . . .

Epilogue

Last—But Definitely Not Final—Words

> IF I HAD TO DO MY LIFE OVER, I WOULD CHANGE EVERY SINGLE THING I HAVE DONE.
> —RAY DAVIES

The following question keeps coming up: "Jon, how are you feeling?"

That's a loaded question. My best answer is that I feel like shit. I'm freaking exhausted all the time. I keep my mind busy focusing on work stuff where I know I can contribute. And I follow sports and do some sports betting. The Mets just started spring training, so I'm cautiously optimistic about how their season will turn out. As a Mets fan, you become accustomed to disappointment, so I never get my hopes up too high . . . even with their recent addition of Juan Soto.

Most of all, I think about my family and my future. Just this week, Mara and I sealed the deal on a two-bedroom apartment on the Upper East Side in New York City that has outdoor terrace space for the dogs. The bathroom comes with a warmed toilet seat and a preinstalled bidet—total heaven for someone with my issues.

The apartment is something to look forward to, and we won't have to face all the Connecticut back-and-forth anymore. Of course, we must sell the house and clear it out—which involves a ton of work I'm physically not up for. But, somehow, we'll manage to figure it out.

In the meantime, I'm going to keep trying to find something that will put cancer in the rearview mirror forever. I desperately want my old life back and miss rock concerts, comedy shows, baseball games, favorite restaurants, and travel—both work-related and personal time away with my family.

Since I'm now on what is probably the only drug remaining that can be used to treat brain cancer, I've accepted that from this point on I will be living with cancer rather than killing it. I don't see the cancer ever fully going away. It's just not going to happen. I know this is my life now. If it does disappear, it's unbelievable—but I've come to terms with the fact that this outcome is rare, given my history and condition. The best I can hope for is to keep cancer at bay and continue to improve my quality of life.

Another thing people often ask: "Has cancer changed me?"

I would say that it has, but not how you might think. For example, I haven't changed my diet. I still detest fruits and vegetables with all my heart and soul. An industrial crane couldn't open my mouth wide enough to get kale or spinach into my body. I still shove bagels and jelly cookies into my mouth whenever I have the chance. I wouldn't turn down Stouffer's French

Bread Pizza if it were placed in front of me. Those things make me happy, so why stop now?

Here's what I think has changed about me: I used to be an angry kind of guy. I wasn't deliberately mean, but I had a sharp edge and exuded sarcasm. Back when I was a commuter, if a rider on a Metro-North train pissed me off, you could be damn sure I was going to rail on them in social media.

The cancer has softened me these past few years and opened my eyes. I look at things from a different perspective. I'm a lot calmer and mellower now and don't get stressed out about the little things. I'm all about just taking it easy and letting things roll off my shoulders.

I never feel bad for myself or ask, Why me? I'm not going to force my burdens on someone else. No matter what else might be going on, I always try to make light of things and put a smile on somebody else's face.

Doctors, nurses, lab techs, and janitorial staff have an incredibly tough job. They deal with life and death every day, constantly hear about everyone's aches and pain, and clean up after messes. The pressure is enormous. Whenever hospital workers enter my room, my first thought is, How can I make their day brighter?

I always try to find a way to make people laugh. Just last week, a nurse came into my room for a routine check of my vitals. Suddenly, my blood pressure shot up over 200. I felt okay, but the number freaked me out.

The nurse kept her composure and said something like, "Whoa, that can't be right. Let me check something."

She put her hand on my heart to make sure everything felt ok. A second later, my blood pressure dropped to a manageable one hundred.

"Oh my God!" I shouted. "You're Jesus! You touched my chest and healed me! It's a freakin' miracle!"

She convulsed with laughter. I imagined her going home that night and telling her family all about this crazy patient who dubbed her "Jesus." I think these kinds of interactions make my situation more tolerable for everyone.

I have room for one last anecdote. With all the stuff I've gone through in hospitals, there have been times when I was in bad shape and needed some help scrubbing myself when showering. On this occasion, three female nurses and a male nurse led me to the bathroom.

All right, I thought to myself, This is kinky.

The thing is: The three women remained outside the bathroom door, while the dude joined me inside. Fuck. My deepest fantasies faded away. It turned out, this male nurse was a crazy, fun guy—but not at all in the perverted way you're probably thinking. He was hilarious and super hands-on, in a professional way. He reached places I didn't know existed and couldn't have been nicer. I left that bathroom thinking I've never been cleaner in my entire life.

As for the future, I just keep repeating the cliché: one day at a time. My doctor probably won't request another PET scan for a few weeks, until he's sure the new medication has fully kicked in. Right now, it's just a waiting game.

I spend my free moments with Mara trying to enjoy whatever little things we can. I finally went home to Fairfield and saw my dogs, Smoke and Lacey, for the first time in months. In the past, they usually ignored me and favored Mara, but this time they showed their love and were all over me. It really hit me how much I missed them.

Mara and I spend our time binge-watching TV shows and films. I often listen to my playlists on Spotify and keep adding to them. The other day I found myself listening to the Clash album *Combat Rock*. It took me right back to my youth. A million incredible memories came flooding back.

With this thought, allow me to close with this piece of wisdom from the great Lou Reed: "My God is rock 'n' roll."

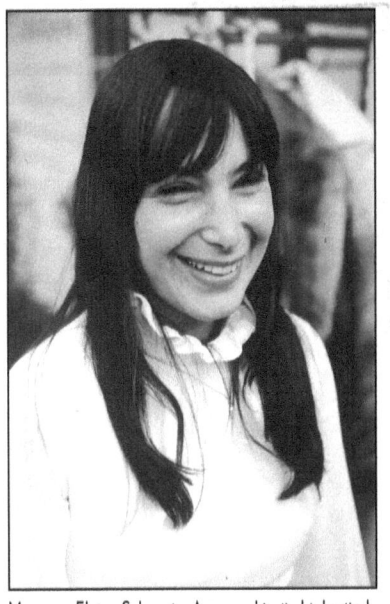
My mom, Elaine Schwartz. Any good traits I inherited came from her.

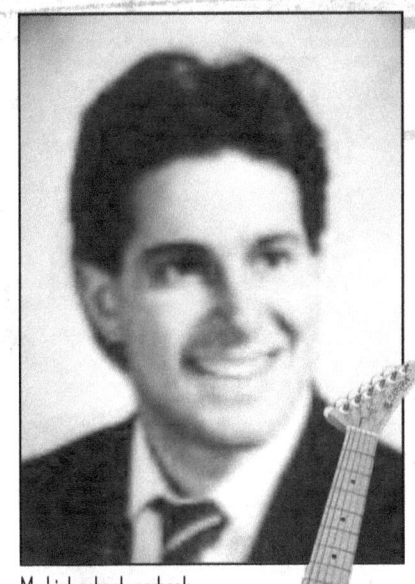
My high school yearbook photo: lady repellant.

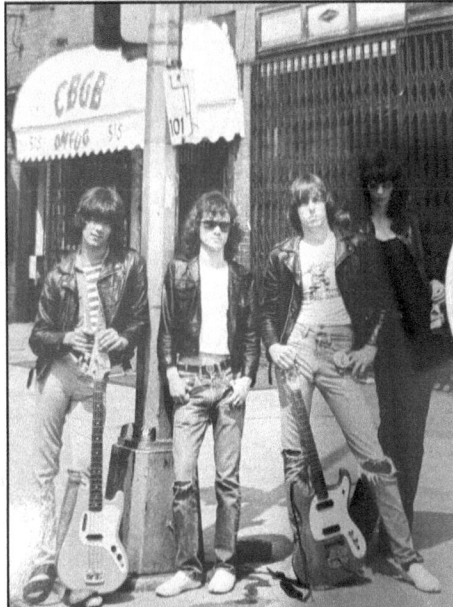
One of my prized possessions: an original photo of the Ramones taken by legendary rock photographer Bob Gruen.

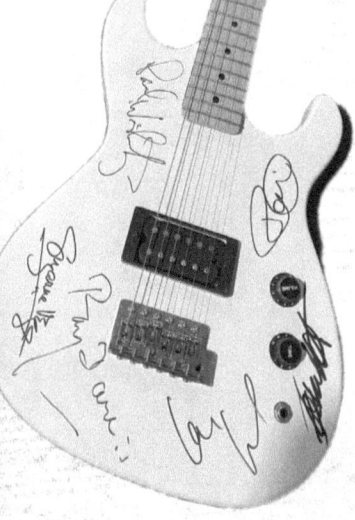
The front of my electric guitar signed by luminaries such as Paul McCartney and Ray Davies. It goes without saying that I don't count Bryan Adams among these rock gods.

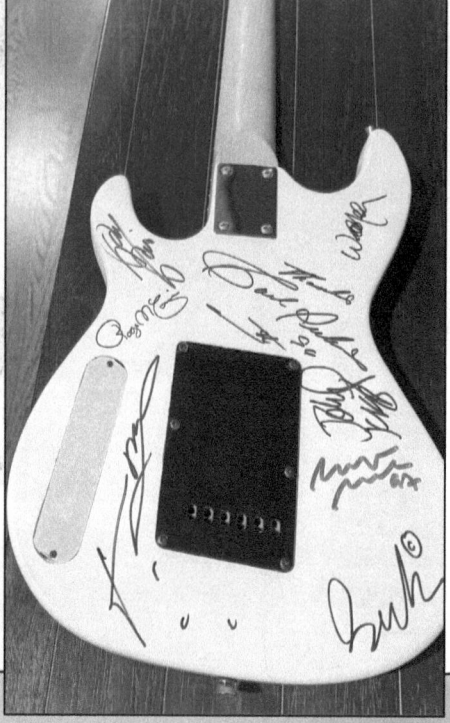

The back of my prized guitar signed by all-time greats such as Carl Perkins and Roger McGuinn. It goes without saying that I don't count Bryan Adams among these legends, either.

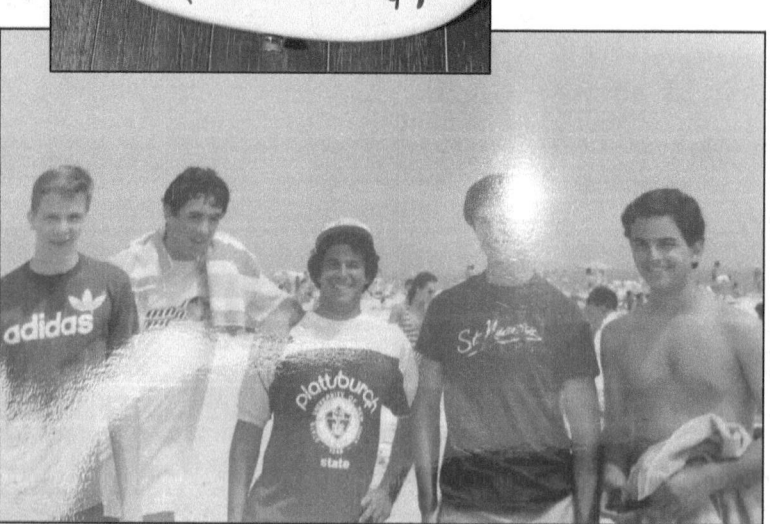

At the beach with my buddies in the 1980s: left to right—Keith, Ed, me, Jeff, and Cabot. The best friends a guy could ask for.

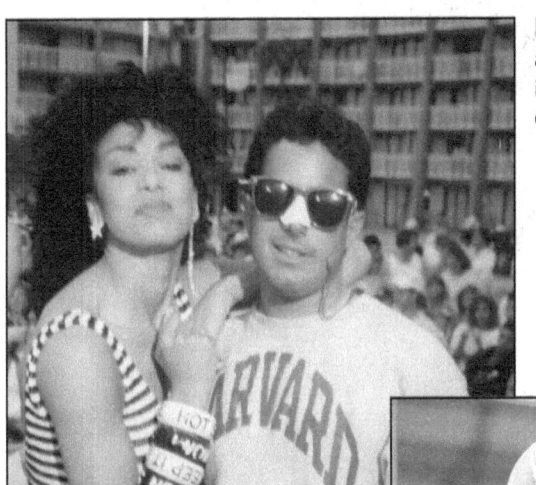

Downtown Julie Brown from MTV and me. I entered a best tan contest in Daytona... needless to say, I didn't win.

Yes, this is me. I would do anything for my directors. In this commercial for Cub Foods, I played the part of a rabid Vikings tailgater.

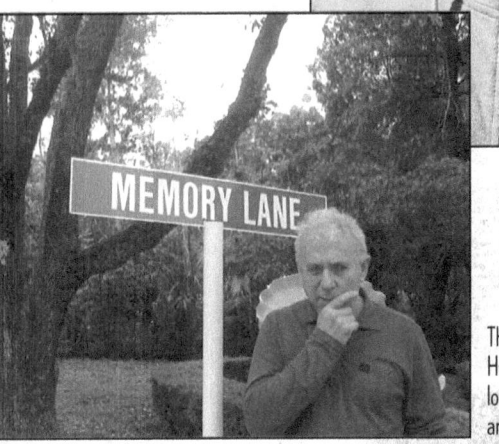

There is only one Tom Schiller. Here we were scouting locations for a commercial and forgot where we were.

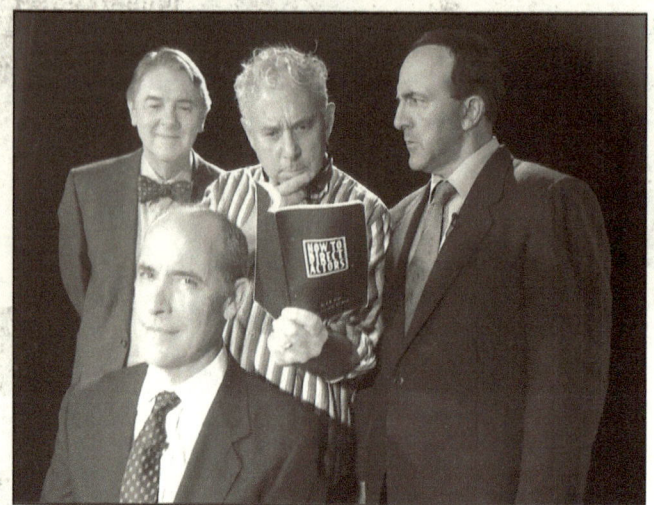

More Tom Schiller shenanigans on the production set for a New York Lottery commercial.

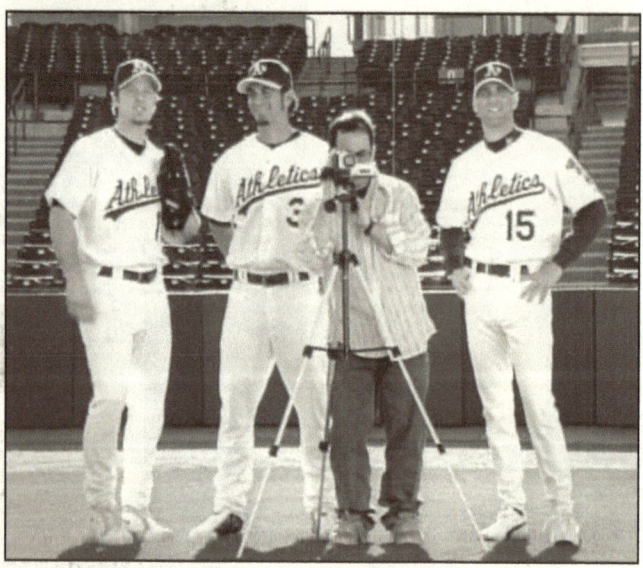

Jonathan Schwartz: actor, videographer, and Major League poser. In this Oakland A's commercial (left to right), I'm sandwiched in between Scott Hatteberg, Eric Chavez, and Tim Hudson.

David Bowie broke the mold as a creative musical genius. His death was a somber day for millions of people and the wreaths piled up in front of his apartment on Lafayette Street. Having him as a neighbor in the Bowery area was a true gift.

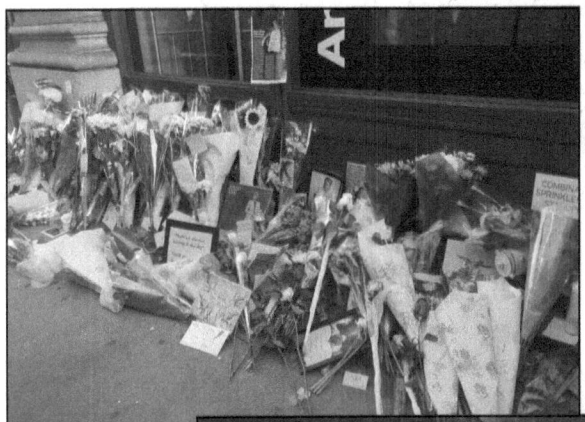

Chris Frantz and Tina Weymouth from the groups the Talking Heads and the Tom Tom Club. They provide a strong link for me between my love of their music and the Warehouse at FTC concert venue in Fairfield, CT, where we all happened to live.

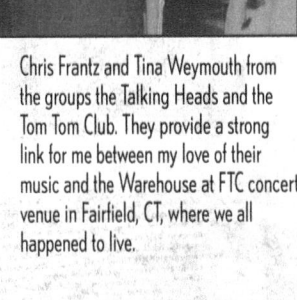

Josh Blum and me: the dream team at Washington Square Films. #raplegends

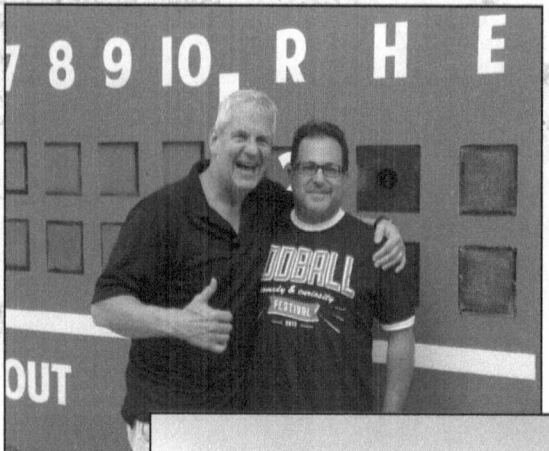

Lenny Clarke was one of the coolest guys to work with. Here we're taking a break from taunting Yankees fans during the Benjamin Moore paint commercial shoot in New York City.

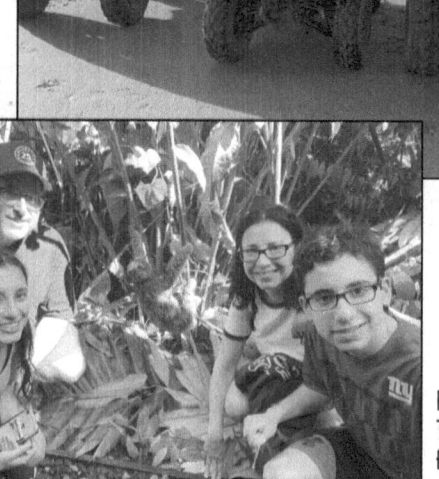

Family times are the best. The Schwartzes attempt to break the land speed record in Costa Rica.

Family outing in Costa Rica. The sloth had goo-goo eyes for me. He knew we were each other's spirit animals.

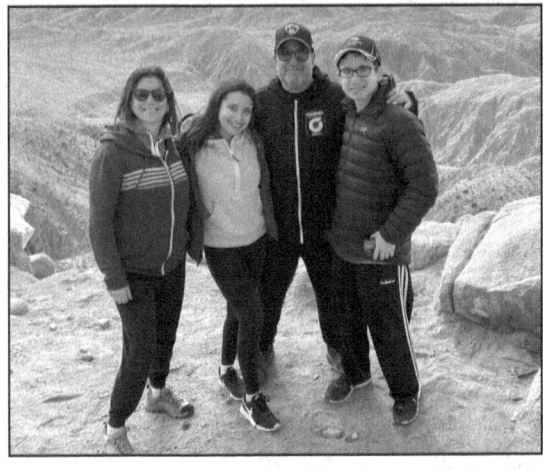

Left to right: Mara, Alissa, me, and Matt. We enjoyed visiting Joshua Tree but dodged listening to any U2.

Mara and me boating in Stamford, Connecticut. During this three-hour tour, she was my Mary Ann.

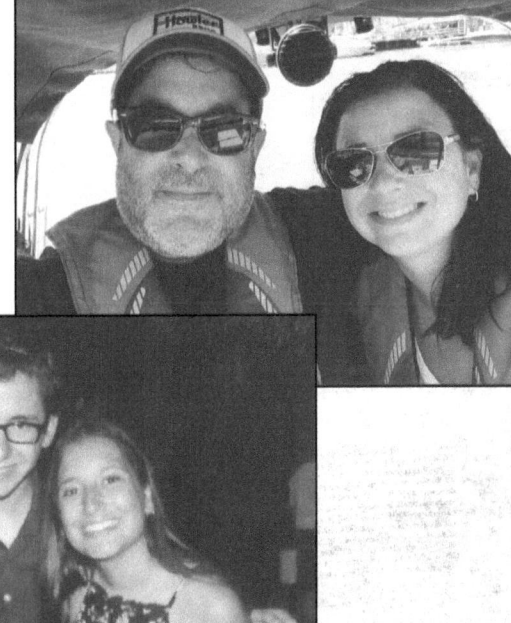

Matt and Alissa partying like it's 2019.

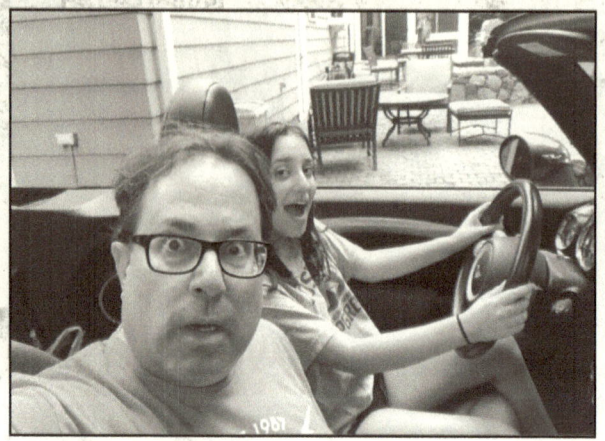

I placed myself in grave danger teaching Alissa how to drive.

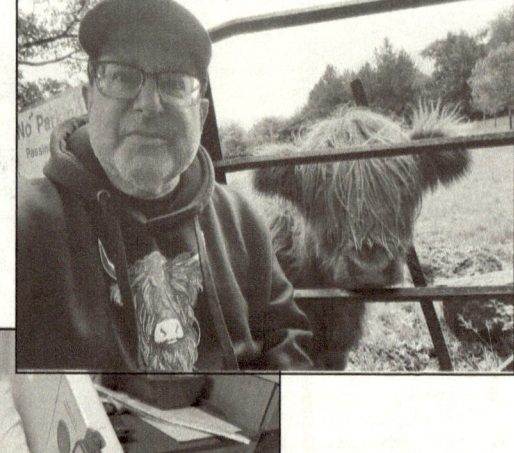

In Scotland posing with a coo, their equivalent of a cow. I really dig his punk hairdo.

Here I'm doing my best Hulk impression. He was exposed to gamma rays. My condition was an excruciating reaction to the stem cell transplant.

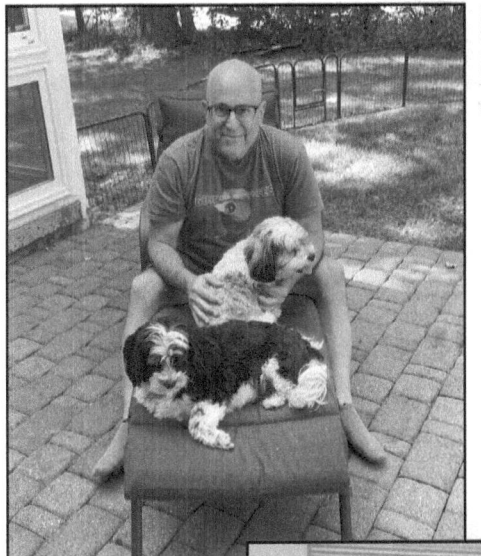

In my backyard with Smoke and Lacey. I'm the bald one, thanks to the chemo treatments.

I get the last word (technically, a flip of the bird) to Bryan Adams. Proudly air guitaring my precious autographed electric guitar on March 6, 2025.

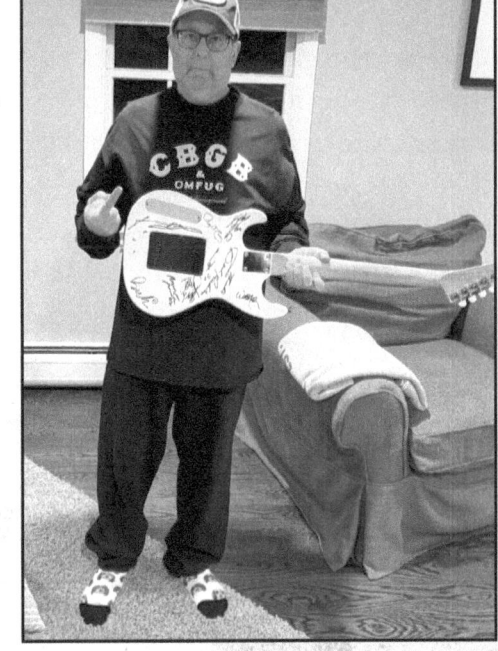

Sources

Prologue:
"If I had five million pounds, I'd start a radio station because something needs to be done. It would be nice to turn on the radio and hear something that didn't make you feel like smashing up the kitchen and strangling the cat."
https://www.goodreads.com/quotes/13513-if-i-had-five-million-pounds-i-d-start-a-radio

Introduction:
"I don't know where I'm going, but I promise it won't be boring."
https://www.radiox.co.uk/artists/david-bowie/david-bowie-in-his-own-words-his-best-quotes/

Chapter One:
"Work aside, we come to New York for the possibility of interaction and inspiration."
https://creativetimereports.org/2013/10/07/david-byrne-will-work-for-inspiration/

Chapter Two:
"Marriage is worse than dying. Why stay with one person for fifty years? We advise against marriage."
https://quotefancy.com/quote/1377569/Joey-Ramone-Marriage-is-worse-than-dying-Why-stay-with-one-person-for-fifty-years-We

Chapter Three:
"I think anger is an underused emotion."
https://www.bookey.app/quote-author/john-lydon

Chapter Four:
"When I see everyone doing the same thing, I want to do the opposite."
https://www.azquotes.com/quote/1328811

"The end comes when the infinites arrive."
https://www.azquotes.com/quote/1134627

Chapter Five:
"I love sports. I love animals. I love kids. I want to save the world. So how do I combine those things? I don't know."
https://www.brainyquote.com/authors/joan-jett-quotes

"There are rich teams and then there are poor teams. Then there's fifty feet of crap. And then there's us."
https://www.youtube.com/watch?v=CDQqjnkThnI

Chapter Six:
"CBGB was a wild place . . . The first time I ever played there was in 1987, I think, with my hardcore band, Scream. And I remember the craziest thing [about] that club was that you could be in front of the stage, and it could be louder than any show you've ever been to in your life. But if you were in the back of the club at the

bar, you could sit and have a conversation with someone. It was the weirdest thing to me."
https://www.azquotes.com/quotes/topics/cbgb.html

Chapter Seven:
"I'm a culture vulture, and I just want to experience it all."
https://www.brainyquote.com/quotes/debbie_harry_267436

Chapter Eight:
"My mind is turning into kind of a fine gelatinous ball of pepper."
https://www.azquotes.com/quote/637968

Chapter Nine:
"Everyone thinks I'm a wimp and even my own band hates me. Oh, well. I guess I'll just flip 'em the bird!"
https://www.azquotes.com/quote/1089687

Chapter Ten:
"There's a bit of magic in everything, and then some loss to even things out."
https://www.goodreads.com/quotes/344832-there-s-a-bit-of-magic-in-everything-and-then-some

Chapter Eleven:
"Cancer softened me up. I like the old me better. I liked being angry. It made me feel strong."
https://www.brainyquote.com/authors/johnny-ramone-quotes

Chapter Twelve:
"This whole thing has become a pantomime."
https://www.brainyquote.com/search_results?x=0&y=0&q=Sid+Vicious

Epilogue:
"If I had to do my life over, I would change every single thing I have done."
https://www.brainyquote.com/authors/ray-davies-quotes

"My God is rock 'n' roll."
https://www.brainyquote.com/search_results?q=Lou+Reed&pg=3

About the Author

Jonathan Schwartz

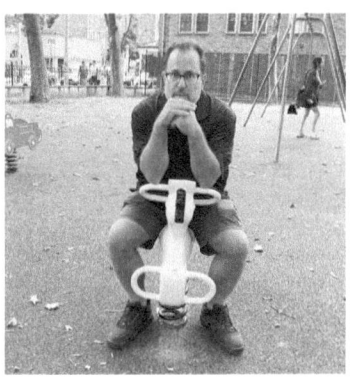

Jonathan Schwartz has been working at Washington Square Films (WSF) since June 1997. He currently serves as Director of Sales & Marketing/Managing Director. He began the TV Commercial and Content division at WSF over a quarter century ago, and it has grown into one of the top production companies in the industry. On the commercial end, WSF has won many Cannes Lions and has been well represented at every major awards show. WSF represents a roster of award-winning directors who create commercials and branded content. Recent clients include GM, Pepsi, Bose, Honda, Chevrolet, Home Depot, Apple, Kellogg's, Popeyes, Dollar Shave Club, Toyota, Amazon, Progressive, Citgo, Ford, Meta, Burger King, and Spectrum.

Jon, who is in the process of fucking cancer, lived with his family in Fairfield, Connecticut, for many years and, as of this writing, is making plans with his wife, Mara, and two dogs to relocate to New York City. He and Mara have two amazing adult children.

Jon only has two regrets in life: he wasn't an official member of the Ramones; and his curled fist failed to connect with Bryan Adams's jaw.

About Grumpy Press

Grumpy Press

Grumpy Press titles have been purchased the world over and translated into one language. Classic titles include *Help! I Pulled My Hammy*, *The Great American Disappointment*, *Are You Out There? It's Me, Jonathan*, *Catcher and the Marble Loaf*, and *Lady Chatterley's Hangover*.

To contact Grumpy Press, send a self-addressed stamped envelope to:

CBGB
315 Bowery
New York, NY 10003

We only accept manuscript submissions written on Smith-Corona manual typewriters. Typos welcome.

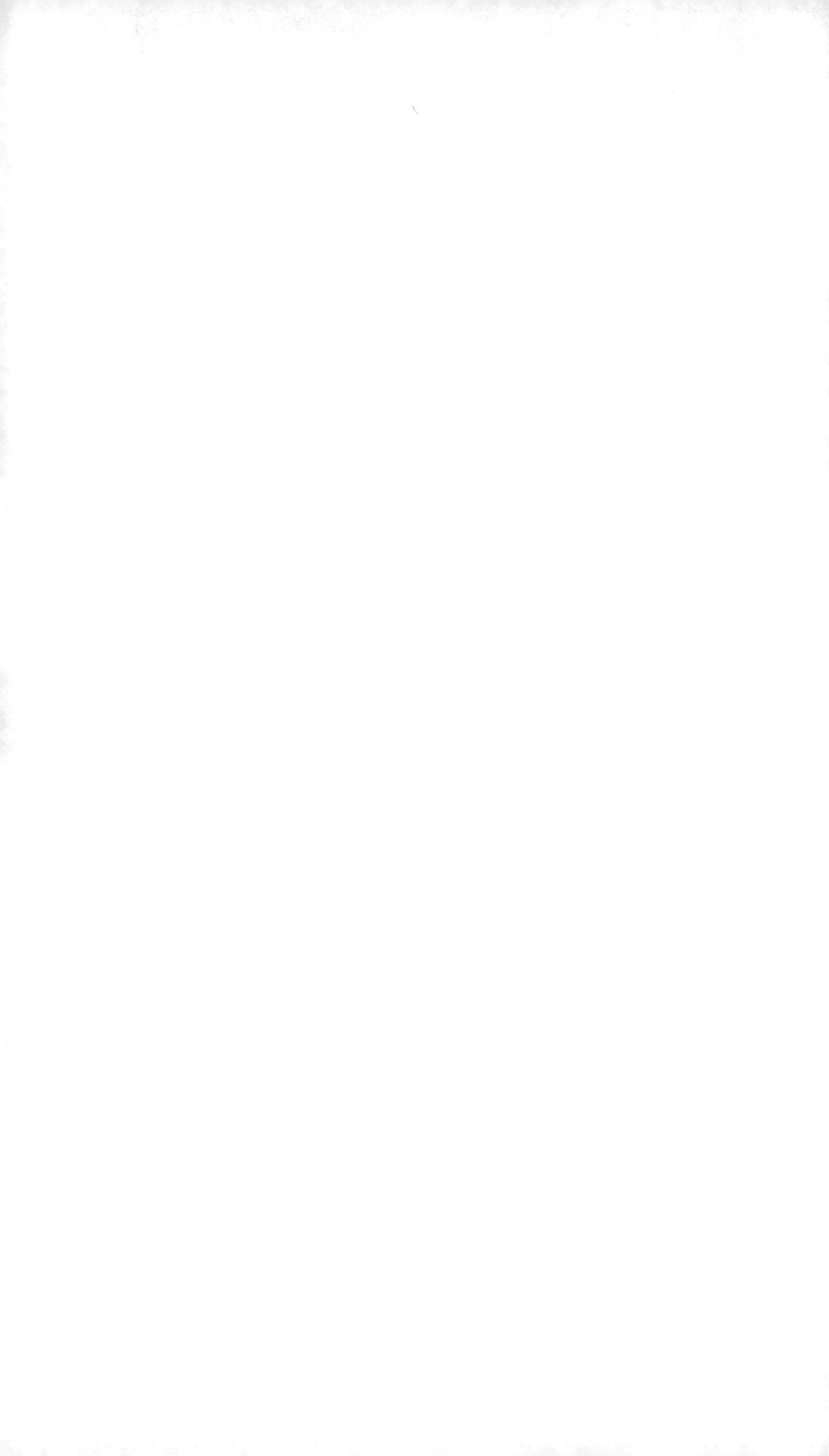

www.ingramcontent.com/pod-product-compliance
Lightning Source LLC
Chambersburg PA
CBHW030242010526
44107CB00030B/1302/J